D1607059

MEDICAL
INTELLIGENCE
UNIT

ANTIBIOTIC-IMPREGNATED VASCULAR GRAFTS

CONTRIBUTORS

Michael D. Colburn, M.D.
Resident
Department of Surgery
UCLA School of Medicine

Hugh A. Gelabert, M.D.
Assistant Professor of Surgery
Section of Vascular Surgery
UCLA School of Medicine

George E. Hajjar, M.D.
Visiting Research Fellow
Department of Surgery
UCLA School of Medicine

Michael M. Law, M.D.
Research Fellow
Department of Surgery
UCLA School of Medicine

Wesley S. Moore, M.D.
Professor of Surgery
Chief, Section of Vascular Surgery
UCLA School of Medicine

MEDICAL
INTELLIGENCE
UNIT

ANTIBIOTIC-IMPREGNATED VASCULAR GRAFTS

Wesley S. Moore, M.D.
Hugh A. Gelabert, M.D.

University of California-Los Angeles

R.G. LANDES COMPANY
AUSTIN

MEDICAL INTELLIGENCE UNIT

ANTIBIOTIC-IMPREGNATED
VASCULAR GRAFTS

R.G. LANDES COMPANY
Austin / Georgetown

CRC Press is the exclusive worldwide distributor of publications of the Medical Intelligence Unit.
CRC Press, 2000 Corporate Blvd., NW, Boca Raton, FL 33431. Phone: 407/994-0555.

Submitted: August 1992
Published: October 1992

Production Manager: Terry Nelson
Copy Editor: Constance Kerkaporta

Please address all inquiries to the Publisher:
R.G. Landes Company
909 South Pine Street
Georgetown, TX 78626
or
P.O. Box 4858
Austin, TX 78765
Phone: 512/ 863 7762
FAX: 512/ 863 0081

ISBN 1-879702-25-8
CATALOG # LN0225

INTRODUCTION

Prosthetic vascular repair combined with infection is an infrequent event. A review of available date suggests that vascular grafts confined to the abdomen, and placed under elective conditions, become infected at a rate of <1.0%. Grafts that cross the inguinal ligament or extend further into the extremities have an increased infection rate that may range from 3.0-5.0%. While the incidence is rare, the consequences can be devastating. An established graft infection cannot be effectively eradicated with anything less than removal of the infected foreign body. Thus, management of patients with infected grafts is associated with an alarmingly high mortality rate. Those who survive operation will have major morbidity with respect to limb loss or organ failure.

In the years since prosthetic vascular repair was first introduced, surgical technique and antisepsis have improved. The appropriate use of antibiotic prophylaxis in conjunction with other preventative measures have lowered the incidence of graft sepsis but unfortunately have not eliminated the complication. It remains a major problem in vascular surgical repair.

The current treatment of an established graft infection has become better defined and has resulted in the salvage of more patients and extremities. However, it continues to be a highly morbid condition even in the hands of experts.

The next logical step, both in the prophylaxis against and the treatment of prosthetic graft infection, is to develop a vascular prosthesis that is intrinsically resistant to infection. The use of such a prosthesis in conjunction with good surgical technique and systemic antibiotic prophylaxis should provide the best combination for the prevention of graft infection. Likewise, the availability of such prosthetic materials would open up alternative strategies for the management of an established graft infection including in situ graft replacement.

This monograph will include an overview of the problem of graft sepsis. It will provide an outline of the conventional approaches used to reduce the incidence of the complication as well as treat established sepsis. Finally, the state of knowledge with respect to the development of infection resistant grafts as well as future directions of research will be detailed.

—Wesley S. Moore, M.D.

CONTENTS

CHAPTER 1

VASCULAR GRAFT INFECTION: CURRENT STATUS REGARDING DIAGNOSIS AND MANAGEMENT

Michael D. Colburn

INTRODUCTION

Infection following vascular reconstruction with prosthetic material is one of the most devastating problems in vascular surgery. Although not common, once this complication occurs, it is characterized by an exceedingly high rate of morbidity and mortality. Recently, the incidence of prosthetic graft infection has remained stable and no further reduction in this rate has been achieved. Furthermore, the complications of graft infections have remain unchanged: sepsis, anastomotic disruption, graft thrombosis and limb-loss still haunt us. Once a prosthetic graft becomes infected, it will almost always require excision and extraanatomic reconstruction as treatment. Unfortunately, the results of these reconstructions are characterized by low patency rates and a significant incidence of infections.

In general, the management decisions facing the surgeon caring for these patients are based on the degree of sepsis, amount of concomitant lower extremity ischemia as well as the general medical condition of the patient. In addition, the location of the presenting infection is important in determining treatment options. Also, a variety of new diagnostic and management options have improved on the clinical outcome of these patients. The purpose of this chapter is to review the current information regarding incidence, etiology, natural history, diagnosis and management of vascular graft infections.

INCIDENCE

The true incidence of vascular graft infections is difficult to quantify; but it is not common. This difficulty is due to the absence of any prospective randomized studies documenting this complication. With the combination of optimal surgical technique and appropriate prophylactic antibiotics, the incidence has persistently been reported in several retrospective series to be between 1-5%.[1-4] This rate is somewhat lower, possibly less than 1%, when the graft location is entirely intraabdominal. This is due to the avoidance of groin incisions. Clinically, these graft infections may present any time following implantation. In two reports, over half of the observed graft infections occurred within one month of operation.[1,4] On the other hand, we and others have noted the manifestation of this complication following an interval of up to ten years.

ETIOLOGY

Contamination of the prosthetic implant is the requisite event leading to the development of a vascular graft infection. The mechanisms by which this occurs are varied and both direct contamination at the time of graft implantation, as well as bacteremic seeding of the implanted graft, have been postulated to occur. Several predisposing factors have been identified as being associated with the subsequent development of prosthetic graft infections. These include: the performance of multiple procedures, emergency operations, and the occurrence of postoperative wound complications such as hematomas or seromas. Multiple procedures allow for the repeated exposure of the tissues to potentially contaminating organisms and may limit local immune responses by the interruption of lymphatic channels and the production of excessive scar tissue. Compared to elective procedures, emergency procedures carry a higher risk of inadvertent breaks in sterile technique and are often performed in hemodynamically unstable patients which may contribute to a relative inhibition in the normal host immune defenses. Lastly, the presence of collections of blood or serum in the wound postoperatively can provide colonizing organisms with a safe haven and adequate nutrient supply to multiply and become pathogenic.

Regardless of the mechanism by which an infecting organism comes in contact with the prosthetic graft, once together several steps must occur in order for colonization and subsequent graft infection to develop. First, there must be adhesion of the organism to the prosthesis. Next, there must be sufficient structural and nutritional support for microcolony formation to occur. Lastly, the infecting organisms must stimulate the activation of host defenses including the development of inflammation and the infiltration of leukocytes. Thus it is clear that prosthetic grafts and colonizing organisms act synergistically to activate the host defense mechanisms which eventually lead to the development of clinically significant graft infections.

CLINICAL MANIFESTATIONS AND NATURAL HISTORY

The clinical presentation of prosthetic graft infections occurs as a spectrum of syndromes ranging in presentation from minimal symptoms to florid sepsis or acute graft rupture. If the developing infection arises in a well healed graft with an organism of low virulence and if the anastomoses are not involved, then the clinical sequelae may be minimal. On the other hand, highly virulent infections occurring in the setting of poor graft incorporation and lowered host immune defenses can lead to severe systemic sepsis or graft failure. Anastomotic involvement typically leads to suture line dehiscence and the development of false aneurysms, hemorrhage or graft-enteric fistulas. Information regarding the natural history of these complications has been derived from attempts at conservative management as well as cases in which the correct diagnosis was not reached until disastrous consequences had already occurred.

Systemic Manifestations of Graft Infection

Fever is not always present in patients with a prosthetic graft infection. However, in a patient with a vascular graft, fever without other explanation must be considered to be a graft infection until proven otherwise. Generalized symptoms of malaise, lethargy and weakness are commonly present but are not specific for graft infection. As with other causes of intraabdominal sepsis, infected aortic grafts can present with gastrointestinal dysfunction. Ileus, nausea, vomiting and diarrhea have all been described in this setting. Petechia on the skin of an extremity, which is downstream from an infected prosthesis, can be presumptive evidence of septic embolization. While this finding is not common, it is one of the classic signs of vascular sepsis. Important laboratory findings include elevations in both the leukocyte count as well as the erythrocyte sedimentation rate. Both these findings, while suggestive of an inflammatory process, are not specific however for prosthetic graft infections.

LOCAL MANIFESTATIONS OF GRAFT INFECTION

The local manifestations of prosthetic graft infections are quite varied and depend largely on the site and virulence of the contaminating organism. A low grade infection in the body of a graft, that does not involve an anastomosis, may be clinically silent. In the groins, induration, swelling and erythema are common early findings. Later, abscesses and sinus tracts can develop and lead to graft exposure. When the suture line is involved, three serious complications which can develop are false aneurysms, graft-enteric fistulas and acute rupture with hemorrhage.

FALSE ANEURYSMS

Contamination of a prosthetic graft anastomosis usually leads to disruption of the suture line and bleeding into the surrounding tissue. When the graft has been incorporated within a fibrous capsule, this hemorrhage is frequently contained resulting in the formation of a false aneurysm. False aneurysms involving the proximal anastomosis invariably go unrecognized and secondary rupture appears clinically as massive intraabdominal hemorrhage. In the inguinal area, these false aneurysms are more easily diagnosed and often present as pulsatile masses which are appreciated on physical exam. Although these aneurysms often appear quite stable; enlargement, rupture, as well as secondary graft limb thrombosis are all known to occur. When a distal anastomotic false aneurysm leads to thrombosis of the graft limb, the clinical presentation is often that of acute lower extremity ischemia.

GRAFT-ENTERIC FISTULAS

The clinical presentation following erosion of an intraabdominal vascular prosthesis into the gastrointestinal tract varies depending on the level of graft involvement. If the erosion occurs from the body of the graft, the manifestations may be limited to continued sepsis and mild intestinal bleeding from the involved mucosa. On the other hand, involvement of the proximal graft suture line can lead to communication between the vascular and intestinal lumens resulting in massive gastrointestinal hemorrhage. Most patients will present with "herald" or intermittent upper intestinal bleeding. These bleeding episodes can occur over a period of hours to weeks and a history of hematemesis or melena in a patient with an intraabdominal prosthetic graft should prompt an investigation into the possibility of a graft-enteric fistula. Untreated, this complication will invariably lead to massive gastrointestinal bleeding, hemorrhagic shock and ultimately death in all cases.

HEMORRHAGE

Free rupture of an infected prosthetic graft is not common but can occur in some cases. Factors which increase the risk of this complication include: poor graft incorporation, open wounds containing exposed prostheses, and delays in diagnosis and treatment. When this does occur, the clinical presentation is dramatic. Immediate therapy is mandatory if any of these patients are to be salvaged. When the involved site is below the inguinal ligament, the diagnosis and control is greatly facilitated. Unfortunately, when this complication occurs intraabdominally, it is rarely possible to intervene in time to save the patient.

DIAGNOSIS

CLINICAL EXAMINATION

The diagnosis of vascular graft infection can be at times straight forward, such as the patient with a draining groin and an exposed prosthesis. Alternatively, the diagnosis can be remarkably subtle, as in the case of a low grade perigraft infection without anastomotic involvement. In either case, the diagnostic process should begin with a complete history and physical exam. Although the clinical presentation of these patients can be variable, several symptoms are commonly present and should specifically be looked for. Most patients with an infected graft will give a history of fever. The fever is usually intermittent and can occasionally be associated with chills and significant diaphoresis. Complaints of malaise and weakness are not uncommon as these nonspecific findings are frequently associated with systemic illness. It is important to distinguish this weakness from that which is associated with significant hypotension. Dizziness, fainting or evidence of systemic hypotension should alert the clinician to the possibility of hemorrhage from the graft and a contained anastomotic rupture or aorto-enteric fistula should be considered. When the infected prosthesis is located intraabdominally, gastrointestinal complaints are common. Localized perigraft infections can cause significant intestinal irritation resulting in crampy pain and episodes of diarrhea. Alternatively, intraperitoneal inflammation can also result in a generalized ileus, and complaints of constipation and abdominal distention have also been reported. Of course, any history of blood in the stools is very worrisome and should prompt an immediate investigation into the possibility of an aorto-enteric fistula.

The physical exam of a patient considered to possibly suffer from an infected vascular prosthesis must be complete both to elucidate any evidence of infection and its associated complications and to properly plan the management. Intraabdominal grafts often are not associated with any signs of infection on physical exam. Specific findings to be noted include the presence of tenderness on palpation, pulsatile or nonpulsatile masses, the new onset of bruits, or any change in the quality of the distal pulses. Patients with grafts extending to the groin must have these areas examined especially carefully as they are frequently the origin of these infections and their superficial location often discloses early signs of infection. Specifically, signs of erythema, warmth, fluctuance and tenderness in the groin are common findings. In early postoperative infections, it is not uncommon for the infection to extend along the path of the recent incision and present as an open draining wound. Frequently, when the incision is opened widely, the prosthetic graft is visible at the base of the wound. Any open wound or draining sinus should be carefully cultured for both bacterial and fungal organisms.

IMAGING

As most vascular graft infections are not readily apparent on physical exam, the use of imaging techniques to confirm the diagnosis is of great importance. Both noninvasive and invasive studies are available for the evaluation of a patient with a suspected graft infection, including ultrasonography, computer tomography (CT), magnetic resonance imaging (MRI), contrast arteriography and sinography, as well as radionuclide-labeled white blood cell scans. Each of these modalities is helpful in establishing the diagnosis of graft infection. As always, the existence of several available diagnostic modalities suggests that no one study provides sufficient information to completely care for all of these patients. In many cases the information obtained by each technique is complementary. It should be remembered that, while all of these studies provide important anatomical information, only the white blood cell scans supply physiologic data regarding the presence or absence of infection. Needle aspiration of perigraft collections, under ultrasound or CT guidance, can provide additional information establishing the clinical significance of an anatomical abnormality identified with these techniques. Furthermore, the aspirated material can be examined by Gram stain and cultures which provide vital microbiological information needed to direct early antimicrobial therapy.

ULTRASONOGRAPHY

Ultrasonography has the advantage of being inexpensive and available at the bedside. It is therefore ideally suited as a noninvasive screening test. In experienced hands, this exam is accurate in detecting the presence of perigraft collections of fluid or air, as well as anastomotic false aneurysms. Unfortunately, the exam lacks specificity and infected perigraft fluid can rarely be distinguished from sterile collections or early postoperative changes. Furthermore, although isolated soft tissue abnormalities can reliably be identified, the full anatomic extent of the process can rarely be determined in sufficient detail. An example of these shortcomings is highlighted by the patient who presents with a pulsatile mass in the groin one year following an aorto-bifemoral bypass graft. An ultrasound exam can reliably detect the presence of an anastomotic false aneurysm; however, it cannot document the presence of infection or completely evaluate the status of the remainder of the graft. Thus, although ultrasonography is a useful technique for establishing the presence of a graft complication, additional studies are needed to determine the presence of infection and the extent of the specific abnormality in greater anatomic detail.

COMPUTER TOMOGRAPHY

In patients with a suspected intraabdominal graft infection, CT scanning is currently the preferred vascular imaging technique. This study is superior to ultrasound in delineating the anatomic detail of the abdominal aorta, intraperitoneal organs, and the retroperitoneum. Localized collections are easily visualized and the status of the tissues around the full extent of the graft can also be evaluated. Findings on CT scanning that correlate with the presence of a prosthetic graft infection include: collections of perigraft fluid or air, anastomotic false aneurysms and the loss of normal tissue planes around retroperitoneal structures. (Fig 1) These changes are most easily delineated when the CT scan is obtained with both oral and intravenous contrast enhancement. Contrast in the duodenum helps define the relationship of this structure to the aortic graft and the administration of intravenous contrast more easily detects arterial occlusions and false aneurysms. It should be noted that perigraft collections of both fluid and air can be normally present in the immediate postoperative period and are therefore not necessarily indications of infection at this interval. Thus, in this setting additional confirmatory studies are mandatory. In general, CT scans with these findings should not be judged abnormal until approximately six weeks postoperatively.

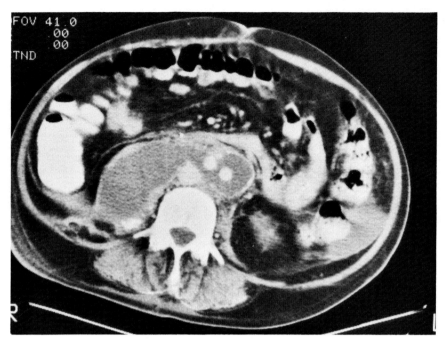

Fig. 1. Abdominal computer tomographic scan of a patient with an infected aorto-bifemoral graft demonstrating a large retroperitoneal fluid collection surrounding both limbs of the graft.

MAGNETIC RESONANCE IMAGING

Magnetic resonance imaging is a relatively new diagnostic technique which has gained popularity for its ability to noninvasively define soft tissue structures with similar anatomic detail as CT scanning but without the use of ionizing radiation or contrast enhancement. Despite the fact that the spatial resolution of MRI is somewhat inferior to CT scanning, its delineation of soft tissue planes is superior and for this reason its use in the diagnosis of graft infection is increasing. MRI can clearly demonstrate perigraft fluid collections and soft tissue inflammatory changes. Likewise, abnormal collections of air and anastomotic complications are also easily identified. In one recent report, Olofsson and associates compared MRI and CT scanning in determining the diagnosis of aortic graft infection in 18 consecutive patients with a compatible history and clinical presentation.[5] The results clearly confirmed the superiority of MRI without contrast over CT imaging in detecting patients with this complication. Again it should be emphasized that, like ultrasonography and CT scanning, currently MRI cannot distinguish hematomas, sterile collections or normal inflammatory changes from infected perigraft fluid.

Arteriography

Of all the available diagnostic imaging techniques, arteriography is probably the least useful in establishing the diagnosis of a vascular graft infection. Nonetheless, biplane arteriographic studies should be obtained in all patients suspected to suffer from this complication. This is because, in addition to documenting the presence of an infection, determining the status of the proximal inflow and available runoff is equally important for planning reconstruction and defining treatment options. Arteriography will also demonstrate false aneurysms (Fig. 2), precisely locate the sites of both proximal and distal anastomoses and identify any arterial occlusions. Lastly, as demonstrated in Fig. 3, arteriography can occasionally establish the diagnosis in the rare patient with moderate bleeding from a graft-enteric fistula.

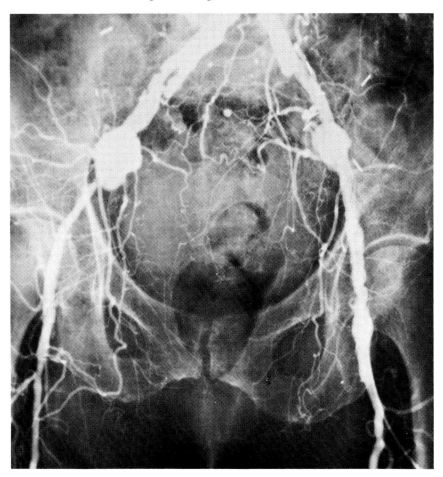

Fig. 2. Aortogram and runoff of a patient with bilateral pseudoaneurysms proximal to bilaterally occluded femoropopliteal bypass grafts.

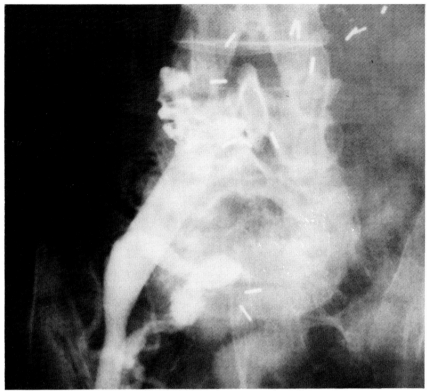

Fig. 3. Arteriogram of a patient with a right iliac to femoral artery bypass graft complicated by an aorto-enteric fistula. Notice the contrast filling the bowel lumen at the proximal anastomosis.

CONTRAST SINOGRAPHY

Contrast sinography can be a useful diagnostic study in the patient who presents with a suspected vascular graft infection and a draining sinus tract. Most commonly these sinuses are located in the groin over the distal limb of an aorto-bifemoral bypass. Injection of contrast material into the sinus tract can document communication of the underlying cavity with the perigraft space. (Fig. 4) Opacification of the perigraft space confirms the absence of graft incorporation and, combined with cultures of the draining fluid, establishes the diagnosis of a graft infection. Although this technique can also provide additional data concerning the size and proximal extent of the perigraft cavity, this information should not be used to infer the degree of graft involvement.

RADIONUCLIDE SCANS

Unlike arteriography or the available noninvasive imaging techniques, radionuclide scans are capable of providing both physiologic as well as anatomic information regarding the presence of a vascular graft infection. The two most commonly used studies are the gallium[67] scan and the indium[111]-labeled white blood cell scan.

Gallium[67] citrate is an inexpensive isotope with a half-life of approximately three days. Following intravenous administration, gallium[67] is normally localized in bone marrow, liver, spleen, lymph nodes, and salivary glands. Abnormal uptake is nonspecific and the isotope is concentrated by certain tumors, inflammatory conditions, e.g., sarcoidosis, pancreatitis, colitis, in addition to infectious processes, e.g., abscesses, pneumonia, osteomyelitis. Several mechanisms are thought to contribute to the retention of gallium[67] by infected tissues. These include the binding of the isotope to inflammatory tissue proteins and leukocytes, as well as direct bacterial uptake. After administration, imaging is usually performed at 48 or 72 hours to permit clearance of the isotope from the soft tissues.

Indium[111] is more expensive then gallium,[67] and its use is somewhat more complicated. For this study the patient's leukocytes are collected

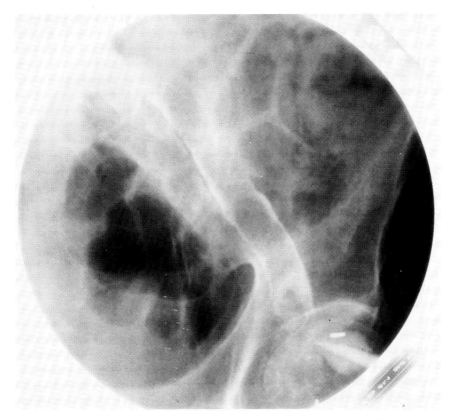

Fig. 4. Sinogram, performed by injecting contrast into a sinus tract exiting through the groin, demonstrates communication with the perigraft space.

and incubated with the radionuclide for two to three hours. The labeled white blood cells are then reinfused back into the patient. Like gallium,[67] indium[111] also has a half-life of three days. However, the circulating labeled leukocytes have a half-life of only six hours so, when performing an indium[111]-labeled white blood cell scan, images are taken 6 to 24 hours following injection of the isotope. The normal distribution of indium[111]-labeled leukocytes is the bone marrow, liver and spleen. Abnormal uptake will occur in any area with increased leukocyte migration such as inflammation or infection.

Radionuclide imaging with either gallium[67] or indium[111] is an important diagnostic tool in evaluating a patient with a suspected prosthetic graft infection. The sensitivities, i.e., ability to find disease

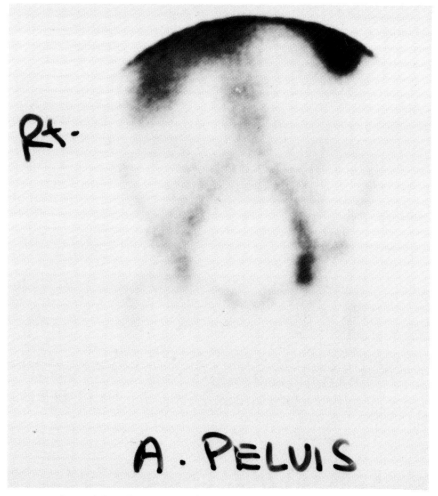

Fig. 5. Radionuclide indium[111] scan showing diffuse uptake along the entire course of an aorto-bifemoral bypass graft.

when present, of each are about equal (80-90%). However, indium[111] has a somewhat higher specificity, i.e., ability to identify disease correctly, then does gallium.[67] This is due to the binding of the indium[111] isotope directly to the patient's leukocytes in vitro, where as the gallium[67] images rely on the nonspecific uptake of this radionuclide by acute phase reactant proteins present at sites of inflammatory processes. Thus in general, in the patient with a clinical presentation suggestive of a vascular graft infection in whom noninvasive imaging techniques fail to establish a clear diagnosis, radionuclide scanning with indium[111] can be very useful and is preferred to a gallium[67] scan. (Fig. 5) It should be emphasized that a negative radionuclide study by no means rules out a diagnosis of vascular graft infection and surgical exploration should never be withheld solely on the basis of a nondiagnostic exam.

One relatively new radionuclide diagnostic imaging technique which deserves mention is indium[111]-labeled human immunoglobulin G scanning. Use of this modality in humans was initially reported by Rubin and associates in 1989.[6] Its efficacy for the specific purpose of identifying patients with a vascular graft infection was also recently reported.[7] In this study, indium[111]-labeled Ig G scans correctly diagnosed 10 of 10 patients with vascular graft infections and identified 14 of 15 patients who did not have an infected graft. Whether more specific detection of focal infections can be accomplished with the use of monoclonal antibodies remains to be determined. However, at least one experimental study using a monoclonal antibody against capsular antigens of *Pseudomonas aeruginosa* suggests that this will soon be possible.[8]

ENDOSCOPY

Upper intestinal endoscopy is the diagnostic method of choice in the patient with a suspected graft-enteric fistula. The endoscopist should most importantly examine the duodenal mucosa very carefully. Specific findings suggestive of a graft-enteric fistula include mucosal erosion or ulceration and occasionally a visible graft surface or suture line. Infrequently the findings consist only of the presence of a luminal clot on the duodenal mucosal surface. In this situation it is important to avoid the temptation to dislodge the clot in an effort to discover the underlying mucosal abnormality. This maneuver can sometimes result in exsanguinating hemorrhage from an aortoduodenal fistula. Perhaps more importantly than establishing the diagnosis of a graft-enteric fistula, endoscopy excludes other causes as a source of ongoing gastrointestinal hemorrhage.

Despite the ability of this modality to directly visualize the entire upper intestinal mucosal surface, it should always be remembered that the clinical experience with this technique has been that endoscopy fails to identify a graft-enteric fistula in approximately one-half of the cases.[9] For this reason, and the fact that this complication is associated with an extremely high mortality rate when massive bleeding occurs, most surgeons agree that exploratory surgery is indicated in patients with an aortic graft and a major gastrointestinal hemorrhage even when the diagnosis remains undetermined. In this setting, a high incidence of unrewarding laparotomies is accepted.

MANAGEMENT

The two main objectives which must always be accomplished in the management of vascular graft infections are elimination of contamination and maintenance of adequate arterial perfusion. In the vast majority of patients, adherence too these principles requires removal of the infected prosthesis and de novo bypass of the infected area to reestablish circulation to the affected vascular bed. Unlike native soft tissues, the lack of vascular connections between the prosthetic material and the host prevents adequate exposure of the infecting organisms to the host immune defenses and limits the effectiveness of parenterally administered antibiotics. For these reasons, complete removal of the infected foreign body is considered necessary to permanently eradicate the infection. Also, because the infected inflammatory process invariably involves the adjacent tissues, wide local debridment combined with extraanatomic bypass reconstruction is usually required. Alteratively, in situ reconstructions with autologous tissue grafts have also been utilized.

Once the diagnosis of aortic graft infection has been established, aggressive treatment should by initiated without delay. Preoperative management includes the administration of appropriate systemic antibiotics. As always, every patient should undergo a thorough history including the identification of important risk factors. Likewise, the physical exam should be complete, with particular emphasis on the vascular system. Atherosclerosis is a systemic disease and involvement in other vascular beds must be identified. The association between peripheral and coronary involvement with atherosclerotic changes is well known and must be looked for. Any patient with a history of coronary artery disease, suggestive symptoms, or silent abnormalities on a routine electrocardiogram (EKG), should undergo a comprehensive cardiac work-up prior to any surgical intervention.

The operative management of a patient presenting with a contaminated vascular prosthesis is determined largely by the location of the infectious process.

Aortic and Aorto-Iliac Grafts

The current standard operative management of an infected vascular prosthesis includes removal of the prosthetic graft, ligation or autologous repair of the involved native vessels, debridement of all adjacent infected tissue, local and systemic antibiotic therapy and, if necessary for the perfusion of the involved limb, construction of a remote extraanatomic bypass through a clean operative field. These principles were first suggested by Shaw and Baue in 1963.[10] Strict adherence to these principles is particularly important in the management of infected grafts originating from the aorta.

Management options in this situation depend on the patient's overall condition and urgency of presenting symptoms. In addition, a determination of the extent of native arterial disease is important in predicting the likelihood of the patient needing remote distal revascularization. As mentioned, arteriography is very important in the preoperative evaluation of these patients and several findings on this study should be specifically noted. First, although restoration of distal perfusion is not always required, this is unusual and most patients will require a revascularization procedure. Therefore, the peripheral arterial anatomy should be carefully examined to determine the presence of any significant lesions which may alter the level or method of reconstruction. Second, the extent of native aorta proximal to the graft and the location of the renal arteries should be determined. This is important in assessing whether there is enough length of aorta to permit graft removal and oversewing of the aortic stump. If the remaining aortic segment is short, or there has been any disruption in the proximal anastomosis, it may be necessary to gain temporary proximal aortic control at the level of the celiac artery. When insufficient uninfected aorta remains below the renal arteries to allow aortic stump closure, the aorta is oversewn just distal to the superior mesenteric artery. Renal perfusion is then reestablished with autologous splenorenal or hepatorenal bypasses.

Once the anatomy is defined and the need for distal revascularization established, a decision to perform the distal reconstruction before or after the removal of the infected prosthesis must be made. In addition, either a simultaneous or staged reconstruction must be planned. Although it has been reported that lower amputation rates and better survival can be achieved with selective staged revascularizations,[11,12] we and others have found that the majority of patients require a simultaneous reconstruction. Performing the revascularization procedure prior to removal of the infected graft has three main advantages. First, any distal ischemia, which would inevitably occur following removal of a critical proximal graft, is avoided. Second, the extraanatomic bypass can be performed sterilely, and the incisions closed and protected prior to contaminating the procedure by exposing the infected prosthesis. Lastly, this sequence allows for the removal of the infected prosthesis without the use of systemic anticoagulation. The disadvantages of this approach are two-fold. First, there is a small but definite risk of the remote bypass becoming secondarily infected from bacteremic seeding before or during the subsequent removal of the infected graft. The overall incidence of this complication is not certain but is probably around 5%.[13] Second, theoretically, competitive flow while both grafts are open can lead to thrombosis of the new graft in the interval prior to removal of the infected conduit. This complication is rarely observed and it is unlikely to be a major problem clinically. Thrombosis in this setting is more likely due to a technical problem with the new bypass. Thus, when possible, we favor performance of a distal reconstruction prior to the removal of the infected aortic prosthesis. This view is supported by other reports in the literature. Trout and associates reported a mortality of 71% (10 of 14) in patients who underwent revascularization following removal of an infected graft.[13] When the remote bypass was placed prior to excision of the infected prosthesis, only 26% (6 of 13) patients died. Alternatively, Reilly et a. who reported an identical 26% (18 of 70 patients) mortality rate when a remote bypass graft was placed first and then immediately followed by removal of an infected graft, were able to further reduce the mortality to 13% (2 of 15 patients) when revascularization was performed first, followed by a staged aortic graft removal four to six days later.[14] This later technique may be appropriate in the patient with a low grade prosthetic infection in whom removal of the graft is not urgent. In the patient who presents with a complication requiring prompt repair, such as overwhelming sepsis or an anastomotic hemorrhage, initial graft removal is mandatory. Distal reconstruction if necessary can then be performed either during the same operation or later if the native circulation is adequate.

Removal of the infected graft should proceed in an orderly fashion. The proximal aortic anastomosis is managed first. An end-to-side anastomosis greatly simplifies this portion of the procedure. When the proximal aortic anastomosis was performed in an end-to-end fashion, care must be taken to adequately secure the aortic stump. The native aorta should be resected back to clean healthy tissue and oversewn with heavy nonabsorbable monofilament suture. In general, the use of multifibered braided sutures is to be avoided as this material may serve as a nidus for continued infection. Lastly, an attempt should be made to separate the aortic stump from the abdominal contents by the interposition of omentum or clean adjacent tissue. The distal anastomoses are then taken down and the arteriotomy sites again closed with monofilament suture. Following removal of the entire graft, all grossly infected tissue should be debrided taking particular care not to damage important retroperitoneal structures such as the vena cava and ureters. The resulting retroperitoneal space should be copiously irrigated with a suitable antibiotic solution and drains should be placed to allow for dependent drainage. Finally, it is important to close the retroperitoneal space to prevent loops of bowel from becoming adherent to the infected and inflamed bed. This can usually be accomplished by the use of omentum or adjacent uninvolved tissue.

Following excision of the infected graft, intravenous antibiotics should be administered in high doses. The choice of agents is based on the results of intraoperative cultures and the known sensitivities of the isolated organisms. It is recommended that long-term oral antibiotic therapy be continued from three to six months postoperatively.

Aorto-Bifemoral Grafts with Proximal Graft Involvement

The operative management of patients with an infected aorto-bifemoral bypass grafts, in which involvement of the proximal portion of the graft has been established, is identical to that already described with two exceptions. First, the approach to remove the graft must also include bilateral groin incisions. Frequently this area will contain dense scar tissue due to the previous groin dissections. A vertical incision is made over the involved groin and the distal portion of the infected bypass graft is exposed with a combination of sharp dissection and lateral retraction. Continued sharp dissection is used to identify and mobilize the native common femoral, superficial femoral and profunda femoral arteries. Care should be taken not to divide any major collateral branches particularly when dissecting around the profunda femoral artery where the lateral or medial circumflex arteries can easily be damaged. When the normal tissue planes are particularly distorted, it is often helpful to begin this dissection distally, over a previously undissected area of the superficial artery, and then carry the sharp dissection of the scarred fibrous capsule back to the common femoral artery. Once these vessels are identified and mobilized, proximal control of the native common femoral artery should be obtained in case it remains patent proximal to the graft anastomosis. The infected femoral anastomosis can then be detached and the native vessels either ligated or repaired with autologous tissue and monofilament suture. Second, when the groin is involved in the infectious process, distal reconstruction must necessarily avoid this area. These remote extraanatomic bypasses are usually constructed laterally to the infected groins; ending either in the distal superficial femoral or popliteal arteries.

AORTO-BIFEMORAL GRAFTS WITH INVOLVEMENT LIMITED TO THE GROIN

Management of contaminated grafts in which the area of infection has been documented to be limited to the groin is controversial and several treatment options have been reported with varying success. Many surgeons still believe that excision of the entire aorto-bifemoral graft is mandatory in all cases.[15,16] Others believe that in selected cases, nonexcisional treatment can often control the acute infectious process and maintain distal perfusion through the infected limb of the graft.[17] Clearly, nonexcisional treatment is only appropriate in nonseptic patients with patent graft limbs and no evidence of anastomotic involvement. When these criteria are met, aggressive debridement of all necrotic and infected tissue, frequent antibiotic-soaked dressing changes and the administration of high doses of intravenous antibiotics can often achieve resolution of graft infections isolated to the groin. This approach has been reported to result in a successful outcome with low mortality and a reduced incidence of limb loss in the majority of cases.[18,19] Also, failures are usually easily recognized and can secondarily be treated with standard techniques. Among concerns with this approach include the likelihood that these patients will require life-long antimicrobial therapy and follow-up as well as the possibility that proximal graft involvement may develop during the treatment interval which could have been avoided had the patient underwent some form of excisional treatment.

Because of these concerns, we have favored a limited excisional approach. If an aorto-femoral graft infection is suspected of being limited to the groin, this critical determination can be made by exploring the retroperitoneum proximal to the contaminated site. A suprainguinal oblique incision is made and the proximal limb of the graft inspected. If the graft limb is found to be uninvolved with the infectious process, then a segment of graft is removed and the proximal and distal graft ends oversewn. Cultures of the excised graft segment confirm the absence of infection at this level. The distal infected graft can then be removed either at a later date, or at the same operation if the circumstances demand immediate attention. Distal revascularization can be accomplished by an extraanatomic bypass in the usual manner. Alternatively, the infected groin can be avoided by constructing a bypass which passes through the obturator canal and the adductor compartment to join the superficial artery in the mid-thigh. If the proximal graft culture is positive, the entire graft must be removed and the same steps described for the management of an intraabdominal aortic graft infection should be followed.

Peripheral Bypass Grafts

The principles of management of an infected distal bypass graft originating below the inguinal ligament are the same as for more proximal grafts. The infected graft should be removed in its entirety and grossly infected tissue debrided. Arteriotomies should be closed with monofilament suture and culture directed specific intravenous antibiotics administered in high doses. A limb which is not viable following removal of an infected graft must be managed by either revascularization or amputation. Frequently it is not necessary to make this determination immediately. If revascularization is required, this can be done using autologous tissue: either saphenous or cephalic vein, or an endarterectomized segment of chronically occluded superficial femoral artery.

In Situ Reconstruction

An alternative method of reconstruction following removal of an infected prosthetic graft is revascularization using an in situ autologous bypass along with surgical debridement and prolonged antibiotic administration. In one study by Brown et al, the survival rate following in-situ reconstruction in patients with aortic mycotic aneurysms was 63% with a re-infection rate of 19% and a incidence of rupture of 11%.[20] In situ reconstruction following prosthetic graft infections has been reported sporadically, and the results have been variable. In a review in 1983, Bunt et al reported a mortality of 56% following in-situ reconstructions in patients with graft-enteric fistula's.[21] More recently, Jacobs et al reported on their experience with in-situ graft replacement in 18 patients with infected aortic grafts.[22] In this study, 12 of the 18 patients were classified as having low-grade graft infections with negative blood and perigraft cultures. All 12 of these patients were alive at a mean follow-up of eight years. The remaining six patients had severe graft infections with positive blood and perigraft cultures. In this group, five patients died within one month of operation and the remaining patient required conversion to an extraanatomic bypass because of recurrent infection. The authors conclude that there may be a role for in situ reconstruction in patients who present with low grade aortic graft infections. A similar conclusion was reached recently in a report by Robinson and Johansen.[23] In this paper, the authors review their experience and that of the literature, regarding in situ replacement of infected aortic grafts. Their findings suggest that the operative mortality of these patients is as low as 19%, and that this procedure may be appropriate in a select group of patients with low grade graft infections. Lastly, Bandyk et al recently reported their experience with in situ graft replacement in 15 patients with low grade graft infections secondary to *Staphylococcus epidermidis.*[24] In this series, no deaths, graft thromboses, or recurrent infections occurred after a mean follow-up of 21 months. The authors also suggest that a reevaluation of the use of in situ graft replacement for infected vascular prostheses seems warranted. In conclusion, when autologous material is available and the bypass can be placed in an operative field with minimal contamination, the experiment data supports the use of in situ reconstructions. It must be considered, however, that use of autologous tissue in an infected bed carries a definite risk of hemorrhage due to destruction of an anastomosis by the septic process.

RESULTS

Despite the establishment of a treatment protocol and the strict adherence to the management principles outlined above, graft infection remains one of the most devastating complications of vascular reconstructive surgery. Overall, the mortality rate in patients with a prosthetic graft infection is 30-40% and up to 30% will require a subsequent amputation.[2,3,25] In one report, 82% of patients treated for an aortic graft infection were dead at five years.[12] Furthermore, those patients who do survive the initial removal of the infected prosthesis continue to suffer from a relatively high morbidity related to their remote extraanatomic bypasses. The best reported primary patency rates for axillo-bifemoral bypass grafts are between 62 and 72% at five years.[26, 27] These studies, however, primarily include patients in whom the indication for bypass was either aneurysmal or occlusive disease. When extraanatomic graft patency is evaluated in patients in whom the primary indication for operation was an aortic graft infection, the primary graft patency rate at three years is only 43% which can be improved to 65% after secondary procedures.[28] Subsequent limb-loss associated with a failed axillo-bifemoral graft is as high as 34%.[28] Furthermore, the recurrence of infection in an extraanatomic bypass graft is significant at about 20%.[28] Lastly, the incidence of fatalities during the course of these reconstructive efforts has been reported to be as high as 25%.[28-30]

REFERENCES

1. Szilagyi DE, Smith RF, Elliott JP, Vrandecic MP. Infection in arterial reconstruction with synthetic grafts. Ann Surg 1972; 176: 321-323.
2. Goldstone J, Moore WS. Infection in vascular prostheses: Clinical manifestations and surgical management. Am J Surg 1974; 128: 225-233.
3. Bunt TJ. Synthetic vascular graft infections. I. Graft infections. Surgery 1983; 93(6): 733-746.
4. Lorentzen JE, Nielsen OM, Arendrup H. Vascular graft infection: an analysis of 62 graft infections in 2411 consecutively implanted synthetic vascular grafts. Surgery 1985; 98: 81-86.
5. Olofsson PA, Auffermann W, Higgins CB et al. Diagnosis of prosthetic aortic graft infection by magnetic resonance imaging. J Vasc Surg 1988; 8: 99-105.
6. Rubin RH, Fischman AJ, Callahan RJ et al. ^{111}In-labeled nonspecific immunoglobulin scanning in the detection of focal infection. N Eng J Med 1989; 321: 935-940.
7. LaMuraglia GM, Fischman AJ, Strauss HW et al. Utility of the indium [111]-labeled human immunoglobulin G scan for the detection of focal vascular graft infection. J Vasc Surg 1989; 10: 20-28.
8. Rubin RH, Young LS, Hansen WP et al. Specific and nonspecific imaging of localized Fisher immunotype 1 *Pseudomonas aeruginosa* infection with radiolabeled monoclonal antibody. J Nucl Med 1988; 29: 651-656.
9. Reilly LM, Ehrenfeld WK, Goldstone J, Stoney RJ. Gastrointestinal tract involvement by prosthetic graft infection. The significance of gastrointestinal hemorrhage. Ann Surg 1985; 202: 342-348.
10. Shaw RS, Baue AE. Management of sepsis complicating arterial reconstructive surgery. Surgery 1963; 53: 75-79.
11. Turnipseed WD, Berkoff HA, Detmer DE et al. Arterial graft infections: delayed vs. immediate vascular reconstruction. Arch Surg 1983; 118: 410-414.
12. O'Hara PJ, Hertzer NR, Beven EG, Krajewski LP. Surgical management of infected abdominal aortic grafts: review of a 25-year experience. J Vasc Surg 1986; 3: 725-731.
13. Trout HH, Kozloff L, Giordano JM. Priority of revascularization in patients with graft enteric fistulas, infected arteries or infected arterial prostheses. Ann Surg 1984; 199: 669-683.
14. Reilly LM, Altman H, Lusby RJ et al. Late results following surgical management of vascular graft infection. J Vasc Surg 1984; 1: 36-44.
15. Seeger JM, Wheeler JR, Gregory RT et al. Autogenous graft replacement of infected prosthetic grafts in the femoral position. Surgery 1983; 93: 39-45.

16. Edwards MJ, Richardson D, Klamer TW. Management of aortic prosthetic infections. Am J Surg 1988; 155: 327-330.

17. Calligaro KD, Veith FJ. Diagnosis and management of infected prosthetic aortic grafts. Surgery 1991; 110: 805-813.

18. Samson RH, Veith FJ, Janko GS et al. A modified classification and approach to the management of infections involving peripheral arterial prosthetic grafts. J Vasc Surg 1988; 8: 147-153.

19. Calligaro KD, Veith FJ, Gupta SK et al. A modified method for management of prosthetic graft infections involving an anastomosis to the common femoral artery. J Vasc Surg 1990; 11: 485-492.

20. Brown SL, Busuttil RW, Baker JD et al. Bacteriologic and surgical determinants of survival in patients with mycotic aneurysms. J Vasc Surg 1984; 1: 541-547.

21. Bunt TJ. Synthetic vascular graft infections. II. Graft-enteric erosions and graft-enteric fistulas. Surgery 1983; 94(1): 1-9.

22. Jacobs MJ, Reul GJ, Gregoric I, Cooley DA. In-situ replacement and extraanatomic bypass for the treatment of infected abdominal aortic grafts. Eur J Vasc Surg 1991; 5: 83-86.

23. Robinson JA, Johansen K. Aortic sepsis: Is there a role for in situ graft reconstruction? J Vasc Surg 1991; 13: 677-684.

24. Bandyk DF, Bergamini TM, Kinney EV et al. In situ replacement of vascular prostheses infected by bacterial biofilms. J Vasc Surg 1991; 13: 575-583.

25. Liekweg WG, Greenfield LJ. Vascular prosthetic infections: Collected experience and results of treatment. Surgery 1977; 81(3): 335-342.

26. Rutherford RB, Patt A, Pearce WH. Extraanatomic bypass: a closer view. J Vasc Surg 1987; 6: 437-446.

27. Hepp W, Jonge K, Pallua N. Late results following extraanatomic bypass procedures for chronic aortoiliac occlusive disease. J Cardiovasc Surg 1988; 29: 181-185.

28. Quiñones-Baldrich WJ, Hernandez JJ, Moore WS. Long-term results following surgical management of aortic graft infection. Arch Surg 1991; 126: 507-511.

29. Reilly LM, Stoney RJ, Goldstone J, Ehrenfeld WK. Improved management of aortic graft infection: the influence of operation sequence and staging. J Vasc Surg 1987; 5: 412-431.

30. Yeager RA, Moneta GL, Taylor LM et al. Can prosthetic graft infection be avoided? If not, how do we treat it? Acta Chir Scand Suppl 1990; 555: 155-163.

CHAPTER 2

BACTERIOLOGY AND PATHOGENESIS OF GRAFT INFECTION

Michael M. Law

INTRODUCTION

The majority of vascular graft infections are caused by gram-positive cocci. While the bacteriology of graft infection varies somewhat by anatomic site, when all sites are considered together approximately 60-65% of reported cases are currently due to gram-positive organisms. By far, the two most commonly cultured are *Staphylococcus aureus* and *Staphylococcus epidermidis*. Coagulase-negative staphylococcus other than *S. epidermidis* are occasionally cultured from infected prostheses as well. Enterococcus and other streptococci are recovered much less frequently. Gram-negative bacteria are responsible most of the remaining 35-40% of vascular graft infections reported in the literature. Over half of these are due to *Escherischia coli*. Proteus, Pseudomonas and Klebsiella account for the majority of other gram-negative infections. Serratia, Enterobacter and anaerobes are occasionally cultured as well. Mixed infections involving two or more different organisms are not uncommon. While gram-positive cocci account for the majority of infections involving the groin and lower extremities, gram-negative rods are responsible for up to one-half of all infections in intraabdominal grafts.

CHANGING PATTERNS OF INFECTION

The spectrum of organisms responsible for vascular prosthetic infections has changed significantly over the past 40 years. The preponderance of *S. aureus* infections in the era prior to the routine use of perioperative antibiotic prophylaxis has given way to infections by more fastidious, less virulent organisms such as *S. epidermidis.* There has also been a trend for a larger number of bacteria to be identified as pathogens. Whether this is mainly due to the widespread use of more effective, broader-spectrum antibiotics or to the development of more reliable and sensitive culture techniques is debatable. Both factors are probably implicated.

In early clinical series from the 1960s and 1970s, *S. aureus* accounted for the great majority of graft infections. In 1965 Hoffert and colleagues reported their experience with 12 graft infections from a series of 201 vascular grafts between 1955 and 1962.[1] *S. aureus* was cultured from 8 (67%) of 12 infected grafts. In the same report the authors reviewed the recent literature (1959-64) and found 22 reported cases of arterial graft infection in which organisms were cultured and typed. *S. aureus* was recovered in 15 (68%) of these cases. In 1966 Fry and Lindenauer reported a series of 890 aortic bypasses and aneurysmectomies over a twelve-year period with a total of 12 postoperative graft infections.[2] Eight of these (67%) were due to *S. aureus.* Similarly, in 1967 Smith reported on nine cases of femoropopliteal graft infections, eight of which involved *S. aureus.*[3] In 1974 Goldstone and Moore reported a series of 27 aortofemoropopliteal graft infections, of which 11 (41%) were due to *S. aureus.*[4] There were a total of 18 staphylococcal infections, and 14 (78%) of these occurred in prostheses implanted prior to 1966, when the use of preoperative antibiotic prophylaxis was initiated at that institution. This report was the first to highlight the significant clinical and bacteriological differences between early and late graft infections. The authors divided the series into infections which presented up to three and a half months postoperatively, and those that presented later; 70% (9/13) of early infections were due to *S. aureus,* while 50% (7/14) of late infections were due to *S. epidermidis.* In 1977, Leikweg and Greenfield[23] reviewed the 178 published cases of vascular graft infection reported between 1959 and 1974. *S. aureus* was responsible for 50% of these cases, followed by gram-negative rods (30.5%) and streptococcus (8.5%). Only 3.6% of cases were due to *S. epidermidis.*

This early experience contrasts with more recent reports in which the incidence of *S. aureus* graft infections has sharply declined. *S. epidermidis* is now the most frequently cultured organism in the majority of recently reported clinical series. Many of these reports highlight the influence of anatomic site and the nature of the infecting organism on the clinical course of graft infections. A review by Bandyk and colleagues of 30 patients treated for aortofemoral graft infections from 1972-1982 revealed that 50% were due to *S. epidermidis.*[5] These investigators also divided their series into early (< four months) and late (> four months) infections. There were only five early infections, four of which were due to gram-negative rods. Late infections were much more common, totaling 25, and 15 (60%) of these were due to *S. epidermidis.* In 1985 Yeager and associates reported a nine-year experience with 14 aortic and 11 peripheral graft infections.[6] While peripheral graft infections presented an average of eight months following surgery, aortic graft infections presented an average of five years postoperatively. Of five primarily infected aortic grafts (not graft-enteric fistulae or erosions) with positive cultures, four were due to *S. epidermidis.*

A wide range of organisms were cultured from peripheral grafts, including coagulase-positive and -negative staphylococci, gram-negative rods, anaerobic streptococci and diptheroids. Edwards has reported on 24 infections from a series of 2,614 aorto-femoropopliteal grafts over a ten year period from 1975 to 1986, in which the greates number of (29%) were due to *S. aureus.* [7] The authors note, however, that in only 7/24 cases were prophylactic antibiotics administered according to the departmental protocol, thus this series may be more representative of the preantibiotic era. This observation is supported by the fact that 63% of these infections presented within three months of implantation. Additionally, cultures were negative in 21% of patients, suggesting that the presence of fastidious organisms such as S. *epidermidis* may have been underestimated. In 1991, Quiñones-Baldrich and Moore reported an 18 year experience (1970-1988) with 45 aortic graft infections.[8] Culture results were available for 38/45 patients. Gram-negative organisms were cultured from 24/38 (63%) of patients, most commonly Pseudomonas (21%) and *E. coli* (18%). Gram-positive cocci were cultured from 21/38 (55%) of patients, most frequently S. *epidermidis* (21%). Of note is the fact that cultures grew multiple organisms in 39% of cases, and that there were eight (21%) negative cultures, again suggesting that the incidence of infection due to fastidious organisms was underestimated.

CLINICAL CHARACTERISTICS OF GRAFT INFECTION

STAPHYLOCOCCI

S. aureus graft infections usually reflect the organism's virulence and invasiveness. They are characterized by early onset, suppuration and frequent systemic toxicity. Extracellular enzymes such as catalase, coagulase, hyaluronidase and proteinases destroy tissue and produce a marked inflammatory response. In contrast, *S. epidermidis* infections are generally indolent, lingering processes which present months to years postoperatively, and are characterized by serous perigraft fluid collections and chronic draining sinuses. Signs of systemic sepsis are extremely unusual.

For the same reason that *S. epidermidis* is difficult to culture, this organism is also difficult to treat. Many strains produce an exopolysaccharide "slime" which forms an adherent perigraft biofilm. This extracellular matrix effectively sequesters the organism from the bloodstream and tissue fluids and thus prevents adequate antibiotic penetration. Slime-producing organisms are only reliably cultured from the broth culture of the graft itself, and this often requires sonication to liberate organisms from graft materials.[9] Until recently such culture techniques have not been routinely employed, and it is believed by some investigators that many "culture negative" infections which present in a chronic, subacute manner may be due to these organisms.

Most strains of *S. aureus* are sensitive to a number of anti-staphylococcal ß-lactam antibiotics, such as methicillin, nafcillin and the oxacillins. This group of antibiotics is highly resistant to cleavage by penicillinase. *S. epidermidis* and other coagulase-negative staphylococci, however, are frequently resistant. Currently, about 65% of *S. epidermidis* strains are resistant to methicillin and nafcillin. This resistance may be mediated in part by altered penicillin-binding proteins. The use of broad-spectrum prophylactic antibiotics since the early to mid-1970s has thus resulted in a declining incidence of *S. aureus* infections and the rising incidence of *S. epidermidis* and mixed infections.

GRAM-NEGATIVE BACILLI

Most gram-negative organisms are of intermediate virulence in producing vascular graft infections. They are currently a frequent cause of early graft infections, particularly in aortic prostheses. Gram-negative infections generally present in a manner similar to that of *S. aureus*, with suppuration and abscess formation. Some gram-negative infections are characterized by a necrotizing process that involves vascular wall invasion, pseudoaneurysmal degeneration, and graft disruption. This is particularly true for Pseudomonas, which has become notorious for the severity and mortality of pseudomonal graft infections. In the Quiñones-Baldrich series from 1991, 3/7 patients (43%) who died perioperatively had pseudomonal infections. This observation has also been demonstrated experimentally by Geary and colleagues, who in a canine model inoculated PTFE and saphenous vein femoral artery bypass grafts intraoperatively with *S. epidermidis, P. aeruginosa* or saline.[10] Grafts were excised 7-10 days postoperatively and examined. In the *S. epidermidis* group, graft cultures were negative (using routine culture techniques) in all cases, although 8/10 grafts demonstrated bacteria and neutrophils on histologic examination. There were no graft or anastomotic disruptions. In contrast, *P. aeruginosa* was recovered from all grafts infected with that organism, and marked inflammation with microabscesses was noted histologically. Additionally, 3/5 PTFE grafts and 5/5 vein grafts were disrupted following infection with *P. aeruginosa*.

MIXED INFECTIONS

Mixed bacterial infections are increasing in incidence. Gram-positive and gram-negative organisms act synergistically and frequently produce a rapidly necrotizing arteritis that is distinctly different from infections due to staphylococci or nonpseudomonal gram-negative rods alone. This synergistic effect has been demonstrated experimentally by Ney and associates,[11] who infected grafts with *S. aureus* and *E. coli* . They observed that mixed infections led to a high incidence of pseudoaneurysm formation, arterial necrosis and anastomotic disruption with free hemorrhage.

ANAEROBES

Anaerobic infections are relatively uncommon. These organisms are more often cultured from mixed infections than isolated alone. Organisms such as Peptostreptococci which are part of the normal skin flora are the anaerobes most commonly identified. The clinical characteristics of anaerobic infections vary with the virulence and invasiveness of each individual species.

FUNGI

Fungal graft infections are extremely rare, with fewer than 20 cases reported in the literature.[12] The clinical course of fungal graft infections is difficult to characterize for lack of a large database. These infections most often occur following fungal sepsis and thus affect debilitated patients on broad-spectrum antibacterial antibiotics who have overgrowth and dissemination of fungal organisms. While these infections may not have a clear propensity to cause arterial necrosis, they frequently result in persistent fungemia and are associated with significant mortality.

INFLUENCE OF ANATOMIC SITE

Peripheral graft infections in general present earlier than aortic infections.[6] The vast majority of femoropopliteal infections reported in the literature present within eight weeks of surgery, with many presenting in the first 30 days.[13] Staphylococci account for a higher percentage of infections in peripheral than in aortic grafts, with *S. aureus* on the decline and *S. epidermidis* and other coagulase-negative staph increasing in incidence. When gram-negative organisms are involved, Proteus, Pseudomonas and *E. coli* are cultured most frequently.

Aortic graft infections present later, in the range of several months to several years postoperatively. There are reports in the literature of infections presenting more than ten years following surgery.[7] In aortic grafts which are completely intraabdominal (aortic and aortoiliac), coagulase-negative staphylococci currently account for the greatest number of infections, approximately 40-50%. The majority of these are late graft infections, presenting more than four weeks postoperatively. Early aortic graft infections are usually due to more virulent organisms such as the gram-negative rods. *E. coli* is the most commonly cultured organism in the setting of an aorto-enteric fistula, followed by other gram-negative rods.

Infections of aortofemoral grafts involve the groin in 70-80% of cases, and generally present as a wound abscess or draining sinus. The majority of these infections, up to 80%, present within five weeks of operation. Early groin infections are caused by a wide variety of organisms, including gram-negative rods as well as coagulase-positive and -negative staphylococci.

PATHOGENESIS OF GRAFT INFECTION

A great deal of debate has surrounded the issue of how vascular prostheses become infected. There are a multitude of possible preoperative, perioperative, and postoperative sources of contamination. It is generally accepted that most graft infections are caused by intraoperative contamination of the prosthesis. The normal flora of the patients own skin is probably the most important source of bacteria, as it is impossible to sterilize the skin even with appropriately timed shaving and antiseptic scrubs. While bacteria are present in essentially all surgical wounds, the presence of a foreign body such as vascular graft material may make normally inconsequential concentrations of bacteria much more significant. It is clear that prophylactic perioperative antibiotics directed at skin flora have significantly reduced the incidence of graft infection.[4,14-16]

Wooster and colleagues studied intraoperative contamination of vascular grafts in 73 consecutive revascularization procedures, 78% of which were elective.[17] Skin cultures prior to antiseptic scrubbing were uniformly positive, and of these 80% grew *S. epidermidis*. In the first 30 patients, graft cultures taken after preclotting were positive for the same organism as found on the patient's skin preoperatively in 35% of cases. This number rose to 56% for cultures taken after the final anastomosis. For the next 43 patients, the surgical team changed gloves prior to preclotting the graft. This reduced the number of positive cultures taken after preclotting to 25%, and those taken after the final anastomosis to 35%. The use of adhesive skin barriers did not influence graft contamination. Clinical graft infection developed in only one patient during the 18 month follow-up period. This study demonstrates the fact that vascular grafts routinely become contaminated with skin organisms intraoperatively, and also suggests that careful attention to aseptic technique can significantly influence the extent to which this occurs.

The presence of a groin incision appears to have special significance in the development of vascular graft infections. It has long been recognized that grafts involving an inguinal wound have a higher incidence of infection than those which avoid this region.[4,18,19] In a series of 664 aortoiliofemoral reconstructions, Jamieson and colleagues reported that the presence of a groin incision increased the risk of graft infection three and a half times, and that the presence of a groin complication such as a seroma or hematoma increased the risk of infection nine-fold over patients without groin complications.[20] Yashar has also reported a series of 15 graft infections in which 5 (33%) of the patients had groin hematomas.[21] Lorentzen and colleagues have reported a series of 2,411 consecutive arterial reconstructions with prosthetic grafts in which 62 patients (2.6%) developed graft infections, and all of these occurred in patients with groin incisions.[22] The highest incidence of infection was in patients who underwent aortobifemoral grafting for abdominal aortic aneurysms (5.9%), while there were no infections in 425 patients who underwent aortoiliac bypass for aneurysms (213) and occlusive atherosclerosis (212). Bouhoutsos has suggested that the incidence of infection in aortofemoral reconstruction can be significantly reduced when the distal anastomosis is placed above the inguinal ligament.[19]

Another potential source of intra- or perioperative graft contamination is the presence of an open wound in the distal lower extremities, which may seed graft material by hematogenous or lymphatic routes. Hoffert and colleagues have reported a series of 12 vascular graft infections in which 75% of patients (9/12) had an open, infected lesion on the distal lower extremity at the time of graft implantation, and 7 of these were on the ipsilateral side.[1] In Liekweg's series, 33% (20/60) of inguinal infections occurred proximal to open foot infections.[23] Lorentzen, in a report of 62 graft infections, described four patients who had distal ulcers containing the same organism which was cultured from the infected graft.[22] Bunt has described the presence of bacteria cultured from a distally infected extremity in the inguinal lymph nodes of two patients undergoing lower extremity revascularization; both patients developed graft infection.[13] Bouhoutsos, however, noted no increase in the incidence of femoropopliteal graft infection in patients with infected foot lesions.[19] In Edward's series from 1987, three patients with graft infections had preoperative cultures taken of distal ulcers, and in only one case was the graft infection identical.[7] The influence of infected distal lower extremity lesions in the development of graft infection therfore has yet to be determined. It is worth noting that while many large series report the presence of distal lower extremity ulcers or gangrene in 20-50% of patients, rates of graft infection remain in the range of 2-3%.

It has also been suggested that preoperative transfemoral angiography may allow bacterial contamination of the arterial tree, and thus increase the risk of graft infection. In 1981 Landreneau and Raju reported 39 wound complications in 1,173 lower limb revascularization procedures which had been preceded by transfemoral angiography and noted that 81% of these complications occurred on the same side as the angiography puncture.[24] Other investigators, however, have not been able to demonstrate an association between prior angiography and graft infection.

Prior vascular surgery has been implicated as a risk factor for vascular graft infection. Dense scar tissue, increased bleeding, and lymphatic leak may all contribute to this phenomenon. Goldstone and

Moore noted that 45% (12/27) of patients with graft infections had undergone one or more revisions of their original graft prior to the development of infection in the same region.[4] In 8/12 of these patients, the infection was in the groin. In Edward's series, 50% (9/18) patients had undergone a previous vascular surgery at the site of the graft infection.[7] Similarly, a report from Reilly and colleagues described a history of multiple previous vascular procedures at the site of graft infection in 40% of cases. Johnson found that prior vascular procedures were not a significant risk factor for graft infection, however only 12/135 patients in this series had prior operations at the site of infection.[25] There also is evidence that uninfected prostheses have a high incidence of bacterial colonization at explantation. Kaebnick et al have reported culture results of 45 grafts which were revised for thrombosis (26) or anastomotic aneurysm (21), none of which had signs of infection.[26] Bacteria were isolated from 90% (19/21) of grafts associated with anastomotic aneurysms and 69% (18/26) of thrombosed grafts. *S. epidermidis* was the most commonly isolated organism and accounted for 69% of the isolates. Slime-producing strains were recovered from 87% of the grafts with anastomotic aneurysm, compared with 33% of thrombosed grafts. No patient developed graft infection following graft replacement despite the high incidence of colonization. This study highlights the fact that organisms of low virulence such as *S. epidermidis* can colonize vascular grafts without evoking the typical signs of graft infection and suggests that colonization or subclinical infection may be associated with the complications of thrombosis and the development of anastomotic aneurysm.

The gastrointestinal tract is a potential source of contamination during aortic reconstruction. Manipulation of the gut may lead to edema of the bowel wall, localized ischemia, and transudation of bacteria into the bloodstream or peritoneal cavity. Cultures of intestinal bag fluid have been reported by some investigators to yield enteric bacteria,[23] while others have found mainly skin organisms such as coagulase-negative staphylococci.[27] In a report on 179 bowel bag cultures from abdominal aortic reconstructions, Scobie and colleagues found positive cultures in 14% of patients.[28] *S. epidermidis* was the single most common organism isolated (n=11), while enteric flora were cultured in 12. None of these patients, however, developed graft infection. Russell et al found only 3/119 bag cultures to be positive in a similar series, and also reported no instances of graft infection.[29]

Likewise, there are conflicting reports concerning the significance of concomitant gastrointestinal surgery in the development of vascular graft infection. In separate series, DeBakey, Stoll and Hardy have reported a total of 670 patients who underwent aortic graft placement and simultaneous gastrointestinal procedures with no episodes of graft infection, leading these authors to suggest that such coincident procedures can be safely undertaken.[30-32] It is notable that most of these cases predated the routine use of preoperative antibiotic prophylaxis. Other investigators, however, have described the development of graft infection in patients undergoing simultaneous appendectomy,[4] cholecystectomy and gastrostomy[33] and anterior resection.[19] These authors argue for a more cautious approach.

The possibility of hematogenous seeding of vascular prostheses as a source of graft infection is an actively debated issue. There are anecdotal reports in the literature of patients with urinary tract infection,[4,22] abdominal sepsis,[4,21,28] and other infections[18] that have developed a graft infection with the identical organism. It is clear from well-established laboratory models of graft infection that intraoperative or immediate postoperative intravenous infusion of bacteria will result in clinical graft infection in almost all cases.[34-36] Relatively large inoculum of bacteria have been used in the majority of such experiments, on the order of one to ten million organisms. Chervu and colleagues have recently demonstrated that much smaller concentrations of bacteria, as little as 100 organisms, will reliably produce clinical graft infection in a canine model when directly applied onto a freshly implanted prosthesis.[44]

It appears from these animal studies that different bacteria have variable affinities for different graft materials, and vice versa. Slime-producing coagulase-negative staphylococci have been found to have the highest affinity for prosthetic materials, followed by other staphylococci and then gram-negative rods.[37] PTFE is significantly more resistant to bacterial adherence than Dacron,[37,38] and this observation has led to the suggestion that PTFE is the graft material of choice in revision surgery, particularly for infected grafts. There is evidence, however, that development of a "pseudointima" occurs more rapidly with Dacron graft material, which may serve to protect the graft from hematogenous seeding.[39,40] As it is impossible to know the true incidence of the transient phenomenon of bacteremia in vascular surgery patients, it remains difficult to determine the actual impact of bacteremia on the development of graft infection.

It is increasingly clear that the native arterial tree does not necessarily represent a sterile environment. Bacterial contamination of vascular prostheses may therefore be, in some cases, inevitable. It is not yet clear, however, to what extent the presence of positive arterial wall cultures influences the likelihood of subsequent graft infection. Ernst's 1977 report of abdominal aortic aneurysmal wall cultures was one of the first to highlight the presence of pathogenic organisms in the native aorta.[27] The overall incidence of positive cultures was 15%, and cultures were more likely to be positive when atherosclerotic disease was more advanced; 9% of asymptomatic aneurysms were culture-positive, compared to 13% of symptomatic and 35% of ruptured aneurysms. *S. epidermidis* was the most frequently isolated organism. Scobie and colleagues have described a 23% (7/31) incidence of positive abdominal aortic wall cultures in patients undergoing reconstruction for aneurysmal or atherosclerotic disease.[28] In 1984 Macbeth and colleagues reported on cultures of arterial wall specimens from 88 clean, elective lower extremity revascularization procedures.[41] Control cultures were taken from adjacent adipose or lymphatic tissue. While all control cultures were negative, arterial wall cultures were positive in 43% (38/88) of cases. 71% (27/38) of these grew *S. epidermidis.* The authors described three graft infections in 335 cases (0.9% infection rate), all of which had positive arterial wall cultures.

Also included in this report was a retrospective review of 22 cases of graft infection for which arterial and graft culture data were available. Fifty-seven percent (8/14) of patients with positive arterial cultures had suture line disruption, while there were no disruptions in the culture-negative group. It appears from these studies that the presence of bacteria in the native vessel may have a distinct association with the subsequent development of graft infection. In 1987 Durham and colleagues reported a series of 172 patients with a 44% (75/172) incidence of positive arterial wall cultures.[42] *S. epidermidis* was responsible for 56% of these cultures. There were six infections (3.5%) over 18 months of follow-up, and all of these patients had prior positive arterial cultures. No patients with negative arterial cultures developed graft infection. The incidence of positive cultures was essentially equivalent for primary and secondary procedures, at 43% and 45%, respectively. Notably, 5/6 of the graft infections were in patients undergoing secondary reconstruction procedures. The risk of subsequent graft infection in patients with positive cultures was estimated at 10.5%, compared to 1.3% for patients with negative cultures. The greatest risk for graft infection appeared to be in patients with positive arterial wall cultures undergoing reoperation. Wakefield and colleagues, however, have recently reported a series which suggests that positive cultures in native vessels may not necessarily be associated with an increased incidence of early graft infection.[43] Cultures were taken of native artery, adjacent adipose tissue, and blood in 84 patients undergoing 75 primary and 9 secondary arterial reconstructions. Twelve percent of arterial and 14% of adipose tissue cultures were positive, whereas only 2% of blood cultures were positive. Coagulase-negative staphylococci accounted for 60% of positive arterial samples, 79% of positive adipose tissue samples, and both positive blood cultures. Over a follow-up period of 1-29 months (mean, 15 months), there was no clinical evidence of graft infection. As most of the positive cultures were of *S. epidermidis*, a longer follow-up period will be required to determine the true impact of positive arterial wall cultures on the subsequent development of vascular graft infection in this group of patients.

The immunologic status of patients with vascular disease may also impact the development of graft infection. Kwaan and colleagues have reported on 12 patients with advanced, fulminating graft infections all of whom had critical deficiencies in immune status as assayed by serum albumin, hemoglobin, immunoglobin, and lymphocyte assays and by response to standard skin test antigens.[45] In this study, 8/12 patients who received total parenteral nutrition had significant enhancement of immune response and accelerated recovery from the graft infection. Of the four patients who did not receive nutritional support, two had a prolonged convalescence and two subsequently died from complications of graft infection.

SUMMARY

The widespread use of broad-spectrum prophylactic antibiotics has resulted in an altered microbial spectrum in the infection of vascular prostheses, with low-virulence, fastidious organisms such as the coagulase-negative staphylococci predominating. *Staphylococcus epidermidis* is currently the most commonly isolated organism, producing insidious, low-grade infections which present months to years following graft implantation. Gram-negative rods account for the majority of other graft infections and are responsible for approximately half of infections in aortic and aorto-iliac grafts. Gram-negative infections present earlier and are characterized by a more acute, intense inflammatory response. Most graft infections appear to stem from intraoperative graft contamination, usually from the normal flora of the skin and dermal appendages. Hematogenous seeding of prosthetic material has been well-demonstrated in laboratory models and is probably responsible for some cases of graft infection, but it is impossible to determine the true incidence of this phenomenon. It is clear that the native arterial tree harbors bacteria in a high percentage of patients, most frequently S. *epidermidis.* The actual impact of positive arterial wall cultures on graft infection has yet to be determined. Systemic factors such as immunologic competence also influence the development of and response to treatment of vascular graft infections.

REFERENCES

1. Hoffert P, Gensler S, Haimovichi H. Infection complicating arterial grafts. Arch Surg 1965; 90: 427-435.
2. Fry WJ, Lindenauer SM. Infection complicating the use of plastic arterial implants. Arch Surg 1967; 94: 600-609.
3. Smith R, Lowry K, Perdue G. Management of the infected arterial prosthesis in the lower extremity. Amer Surg 1967; 33: 711-714.
4. Goldstone J, Moore WS. Infection in vascular prostheses: Clinical manifestations and surgical management. Am J Surg 1974; 128: 225-233.
5. Bandyk D, Berni G, Thiele B, Towne J. Aortofemoral graft infection due to *Staphylococcous epidermidis.* Arch Surg 1984; 119: 102-108.
6. Yeager R, McConnell D, Sasaki T, Vetto R. Aortic and peripheral prosthetic graft infection: Differential management and causes of mortality. Am J Surg 1985; 150: 36-41.
7. Edwards W, Martin R, Jenkins J et al. Primary graft infections. J Vasc Surg 1987; 6: 235-239.
8. Quiñones-Baldrich WJ, Hernandez JJ, Moore WS. Long-term results following surgical management of aortic graft infection. Arch Surg 1991; 126: 507-511.
9. Tollefson D, Bandyk D, Kaebnick H et al. Surface biofilm disruption: enhanced recovery of microorganisms from vascular prostheses. Arch Surg 1987; 122: 38-43.
10. Geary K, Tomkiewicz Z, Harrison H et al. Differential effects of a gram-negative and a gram-positive infection on autogenous and prosthetic grafts. J Vasc Surg 1990; 11: 339-347.
11. Ney AL, Kelly PH, Tsukayama DT, Bubrick MP. Fibrin glue-antibiotic suspension in the prevention of prosthetic graft infection. The Journal of Trauma 1990; 30(8): 1000-1006.
12. Doscher W, Krishnasastry K, Deckoff S. Fungal graft infections: case report and review of the literature. J Vasc Surg 1987; 6: 398-402.
13. Bunt TJ, Mohr J. Incidence of positive inguinal lymph node cultures during peripheral revascularization. American Journal of Surgery 1984; 50: 522-523.
14. Kaiser A, Clayson K, Mulberin J. Antibiotic prophylaxis in vascular surgery. Ann Surg 1976; 188: 283-289.
15. Salzmann G. Perioperative infection prophylaxis in vascular surgery: A randomized prospective study. Thorac Cardiovasc Surg 1983; 31: 239-242.
16. Hasselgren P, Ivarsson L, Risberg B, Seeman T. Effects of prophylactic antibiotics in vascular surgery. Ann Surg 1984; 200: 86-92.
17. Wooster D, Louch R, Kradjen S. Intraoperative bacterial contamination of vascular

grafts: a prospective study. Can J Surg 1985; 28: 407-409.

18. Szilagyi DE, Smith RF, Elliott JP, Vrandecic MP. Infection in arterial reconstruction with synthetic grafts. Ann Surg 1972; 176: 321-323.

19. Bouhoutsos J, Chavatsas D, Martin P, Morris T. Infected synthetic arterial grafts. Br J Surg 1974; (61): 108-111.

20. Jamieson G, DeWeese J, Rob C. Infected arterial grafts. Ann Surg 1975; 181: 850-852.

21. Yashar J, Weyman A, Burnard R, Yashar J. Survival and limb salvage in patients with infected arterial prostheses. Am J Surg 1978; 135: 499-504.

22. Lorentzen JE, Nielsen OM, Arendrup H. Vascular graft infection: an analysis of 62 graft infections in 2411 consecutively implanted synthetic vascular grafts. Surgery 1985; 98: 81-86.

23. Liekweg WG, Greenfield LJ. Vascular prosthetic infections: Collected experience and results of treatment. Surgery 1977; 81(3): 335-342.

24. Landreneau M, Raju S. Infections after elective bypass surgery for lower limb ischemia: The influence of preoperative transcutaneous arteriography. Surgery 1981; 90: 956-961.

25. Johnson JA, Cogbill TH, Strutt PJ, Gundersen AL. Wound complications after infrainguinal bypass. Classification, predisposing factors, and management. Arch Surg 1988; 123: 859-862.

26. Kaebnick H, Bandyk D, Bergamini T, Towne J. The microbiology of explanted vascular prostheses. Surgery 1987; 102: 756-761.

27. Ernst C, Campbell H, Daugherty M et al. Incidence and significance of intraoperative bacterial cultures during abdominal aortic aneurysmectomy. Ann Surg 1977; 185: 626-633.

28. Scobie K, McPhail N, Barber G, Elder R. Bacteriologic monitoring in abdominal aortic surgery. Can J Surg 1979; 22: 368-371.

29. Russell H, Barnes R, Baker W. Sterility of intestinal transudate during aortic reconstructive procedures. Arch Surg 1975; 110: 402-404.

30. DeBakey M, Ochsner J, Cooley D. Associated intraabdominal lesions encountered during resection of aortic aneurysms: surgical considerations. Dis Colon Rectum 1960; (3): 485-489.

31. Stoll W. Surgery for intraabdominal lesions associated with resection of aortic aneurysms. Wis Med J 1966; 65: 89-90.

32. Hardy J, Tompkins W, Chavez C, Conn J. Combining intra-abdominal arterial grafting with gastrointestinal or biliary tract procedure. Am J Surg 1973; 126: 598-600.

33. Becker R, Blundell P. Infected aortic bifurcation grafts: experience with 14 patients. Surgery 1976; 80: 544-549.

34. Moore WS, Chvapil M, Sieffert G, Keown K. Development of an infection resistant vascular prosthesis. Arch Surg 1981; 116: 1403-1407.

35. White J, Benvenisty A, Reemtsma K et al. Simple methods for direct antibiotic protection of synthetic vascular grafts. J Vasc Surg 1984; 1: 372-380.

36. Chervu A, Moore WS, Gelabert HA et al. Prevention of graft infection by use of prostheses bonded with a rifampin/collagen release system. J Vasc Surg 1991; 14(4): 521-525.

37. Schmitt D, Bandyk D, Pequet A, Towne J. Bacterial adherence to vascular prostheses.

J Vasc Surg 1986; 3: 732-740.

38. Rosenman J, Pearce W, Kempczinski R. Bacterial adherence to vascular grafts after in vitro bacteremia. J Surg Res 1985; 38: 648-655.

39. Malone JM, Moore WS, Campagna G, Bean B. Bacteremic infectability of vascular grafts: The influence of pseudointimal integrity and duration of graft infection. Surgery 1975; 78: 211-216.

40. Moore WS, Malone JM, Keown K. Prosthetic arterial graft material. Influence on neointimal healing and bacteremic infectibility. Arch Surg 1980; 115: 1379-1383.

41. Macbeth G, Rubin J, McIntyre K, J G, Malone J. The relevance of arterial wall microbiology to the treatment of prosthetic graft infections: Graft infection vs arterial infection. J Vasc Surg 1984; 1: 750-756.

42. Durham J, Malone J, Bernhard V. The impact of multiple operations on the importance of arterial wall cultures. J Vasc Surg 1987; 5: 160-169.

43. Wakefield T, Pierson C, Schaberg D et al. Artery, periarterial adipose tissue, and blood microbiology during vascular reconstructive surgery: Perioperative and early postoperative observations. J Vasc Surg 1990; 11: 624-628.

44. Chervu A et al. J Vasc Surg (in press).

45. Kwaan JHM, Dahl RK, Connolly J. Immunocompetence in patients with prosthetic graft infection. J Vasc Surg 1984; 1: 45-49.

CLINICAL AND EXPERIMENTAL USE OF ANTIBIOTICS IN THE PROPHYLAXIS OF GRAFT INFECTIONS

Michael M. Law

PENICILLINS

Discovered in 1928 and first administered to patients in 1941, the penicillins remain an extremely important part of modern antibacterial therapy. Their broad spectrum of activity and the unique characteristics of the penicillin subgroups make them invaluable in a wide variety of infectious processes. Penicillins are composed of adjoining ß-lactam and thiazolidine rings to which is attached a side chain. (Fig. 1) The ß-lactam ring is essential for antimicrobial activity, while the side chain confers the pharmacokinetic properties and antibacterial spectrum of individual penicillins. Any alteration of the ß-lactam ring generally renders a penicillin inactive. Penicillin G is a fermentation product of the mold *Penicillium notatum* and is the only natural penicillin in clinical use. All others are semisynthetic derivatives of the parent compound 6-aminopenicillanic acid.

The penicillins are inhibitors of bacterial cell wall biosynthesis. They inhibit the formation of peptidoglycan by interfering with cross-linking of peptidoglycan precursors. Peptidoglycan is a polymer of glycan chains cross-linked by peptide chains, which provides the cell wall with rigidity and stability. Penicillins inhibit the membrane-bound transpeptidase enzyme which completes the cross-linking process. There is evidence, however, that the actual lethal event is activation

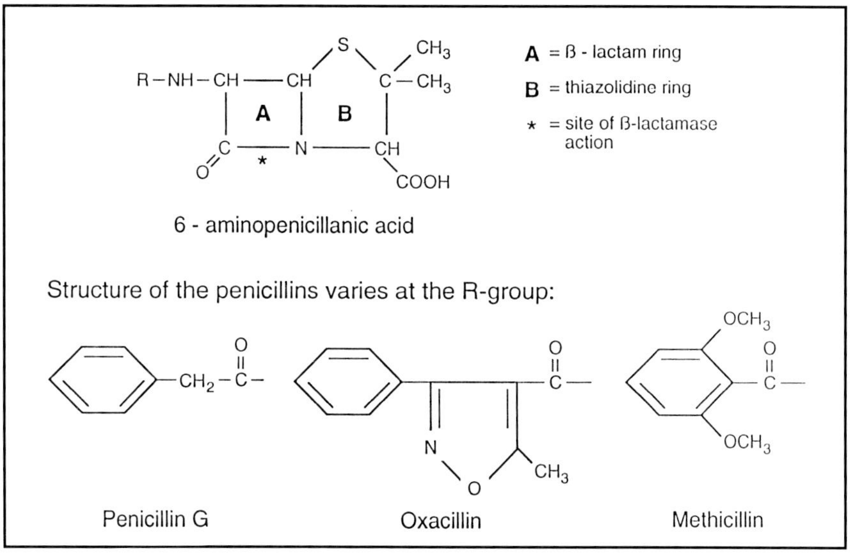

Fig. 1. PENICILLINS

of cell wall proteins called autolysins, which normally provide the necessary gaps of cell wall-membrane growth points.[1] As well, there appear to be additional mechanisms of action which are important in gram-negative organisms, which have an extremely attenuated cell wall. Multiple proteins are associated with the cell wall which bind pencillins and are directly involved with maintaining its structural integrity. Interference with the function of these proteins can produce shape changes and delayed lysis.[1,2]

Bacteria may be intrinsically resistant to the penicillins due to structural differences in their penicillin-binding proteins or because of a given antibiotic's inability to penetrate to its site of action. The latter is influenced by the nature of the side-chain molecule. Many bacteria produce ß-lactamases, which hydrolyze the ß-lactam ring and inactivate penicillin antibiotics. This mechanism of resistance is clinically the most important and is present in both gram-positive and gram-negative organisms. Within 15 years of the introduction of penicillin G, over half of all staphylococcal isolates were resistant in this manner. This promoted the development of the ß-lactamase-stable anti-staphylococcal penicillins. The ß-lactamase of gram-positive organisms is plasmid-encoded, inducible and secreted in large amounts into the extracellular space. In gram-negative organisms it may be encoded on chromosomes or plasmids, may be constitutive or inducible and is produced in small amounts in the space between the inner and outer cell membranes where the enzymes of peptidoglycan synthesis are located.[2] Inhibitors of ß-lactamase have been developed for administration with penicillins in an effort to overcome this problem. Clavulanic acid and sulbactam each contain a ß-lactam ring and act as competitive inhibitors of ß-lactamase.

Penicillin antibiotics are grouped according to their antibacterial spectrum, which is determined by the nature of the side chain molecule. Penicillin G and V are highly active against gram-positive cocci, but are quite susceptible to inactivation by ß-lactamase. Penicillin G is also active against a number of anaerobes. The ß-lactamase-resistant penicillins (methicillin, nafcillin, oxacillin, cloxacillin and dicloxacillin) are highly active against staphylococci which produce this enzyme. A third group of penicillins including ampicillin and amoxicillin has a spectrum of activity extended to include some gram-negative rods such as *E. coli*. Carbenicillin and ticarcillin are extended to include Pseudomonas and piperacillin and mezlocillin have an antibacerial spectrum extended still further to include Klebsiella, Enterobacter and others. These antibiotics are referred to as the broad-spectrum or antipseudomonal penicillins.

The pharmacokinetic properties of the penicillins also vary according to the nature of the side chain. Most are relatively hydrophilic and are widely distributed in various body fluids.[3] Penicillin G and methicillin are rapidly excreted in unchanged form by the kidneys, while the oxacillins and nafcillin undergo hepatic metabolism. Adverse reactions are mainly hypersensitivity reactions, with a reported incidence of 0.7-10%.[4] While most consist of fever, urticaria and edema, anaphylaxis may occur.

CLINICAL AND EXPERIMENTAL USE

Although historically the penicillins have been widely used as prophylactic agents in vascular surgery, the cephalosporins have essentially supplanted them as the agents of choice for this indication. While there are a number of clinical reports which indicate that these two classes of antibiotics have equal efficacy in the prevention of postoperative graft infection[5,6], the cephalosporins are generally more ß-lactamase-resistant and have a lower incidence of severe hypersensitivity reactions.

The penicillins have been studied extensively in ongoing efforts to develop an antibiotic-impregnated, infection-resistant vascular prosthesis. A technique for the ionic bonding of anionic antibiotics to polytetrafluoroethylene graft material using cationic surfactant agents was developed over a decade ago by Henry, Harvey, Jagpal and Greco.[7,8] Initial in vitro studies and an in vivo model involving the subcutaneous placement of graft material in rats indicated that treated grafts might be effective in the prophylaxis and treatment of vascular graft infections.[9,10,11] In 1980 Greco et al reported that oxacillin-bonded PTFE aortic grafts which were implanted in six dogs and contaminated intraoperatively with S. *aureus* were found to be infection-resistant compared to six untreated PTFE controls.[12] When harvested at six weeks the treated grafts were found to have fewer bacteria in the graft matrix on histologic examination (1 versus 5), improved patency (6 versus 1) and better host survival (6 versus 2). There were three treated and five untreated grafts which were culture-positive for *S. aureus,* and this difference was not statistically significant. Although this study involved small cohorts, it demonstrated that an ionically-bonded penicillin antibiotic could be effective *in* vivo in protecting a graft contaminated with a large number of bacteria at the time of implantation. This finding was confirmed in a similar experiment involving larger cohorts.[13] A subsequent report from this group, using the same model, demonstrated that PTFE grafts with ionically-bonded oxacillin were extremely effective in eradicating bacteria and in maintaining graft patency, as compared to untreated and antibiotic-soaked (but not bonded) controls.[14] Grafts merely soaked in oxacillin fared no better than the untreated controls. Among the oxacillin-bonded grafts only 2/40 graft and site cultures were positive, while 33/40 graft and site cultures were positive in the untreated and antibiotic-soaked groups.

Having demonstrated the efficacy of such grafts in a model of intraoperative contamination, Greco and colleagues then took the issue a step farther by using antibiotic-bonded grafts in a model of established vascular graft infection.[15] Forty dogs underwent placement of an infrarenal aortic graft and intraoperative contamination with *S. aureus* as in previous experiments. Reoperation was performed upon detection of elevated temperature or leukocyte count, positive blood cultures or at the end of three weeks; at which time the infected graft was removed and replaced with either an untreated graft or one bonded with penicillin G in one of two solvents. Thirteen animals were excluded due to death or to lack of active graft infection. The replacement grafts were harvested at three weeks. Penicillin-bonded grafts were found to have significantly fewer positive graft cultures (1/9 and 2/9 for each solvent) compared to the untreated control grafts (8/9). All grafts bonded with benzylalkonium remained patent while 4/9 bonded with tridodecyl-methylammonium chloride (TDMAC) and 3/9 control grafts had occluded, suggesting that TDMAC is thrombogenic and therefore an undesirable solvent for antibiotic bonding. In a separate experiment involving the placement of grafts coated in these two solvents in rat muscle pouches, the authors were able to demonstrate that such grafts absorb significant amounts of parenterally-administered penicillin G, suggesting that surfactant-treated grafts can be "recharged" with antibiotic at a time distant from implantation. Although it has not been demonstrated that surfactant-treated graft materials retain this property over time, the possibility of concentrating parenterally administered antibiotics at the site of graft infection is appealing.

In 1988 this group reported the successful use of Dacron grafts with surfactant-bonded oxacillin in their canine model of intraoperative graft infection.[16] At three weeks following surgery only 30% of the antibiotic-bonded grafts were infected, compared to 90% of controls and 80% of animals who received pre- and intraoperative parenteral antibiotics. Antibiotic-bonded grafts were also superior in terms of patency with 9/10 grafts open at the time of explantation, versus 5/10 untreated controls and 4/10 which received parenteral antibiotics only.

As the majority of vascular graft infections are caused by staphylococci, an anti-staphylococcal penicillin such as oxacillin would seem to be a more appropriate prophylactic agent than the relatively ß-lactamase-sensitive penicillin G. While the emergence of bacterial resistance may not be as great an issue in prophylaxis as it is in ongoing infection, and penicillin G has been proven effective in an animal model of established infection involving a sensitive strain of *S. aureus*, more than 90% of *S. aureus* and most strains of *S. epidermidis* isolated in or outside of hospitals are now resistant to penicillin G.[2] This consideration is of particular importance if antibiotic-bonded grafts are to be used in the replacement of infected grafts. Accordingly, most investigators have focused on oxacillin as the ideal penicillin antibiotic for bonding to prosthetic grafts.

Other investigators have described promising results with penicillin-bonded vascular grafts. In 1984 White and colleagues reported the incorporation of the highly protein-bound antibiotics nafcillin, cefazolin and cefamandole into Dacron grafts by adding them to the blood used to preclot the grafts.[17] The antibiotics became incorporated into the fibrin-protein matrix, and remained on the grafts for up to 96 hours in an in vitro elution experiment. In the same report, the use of silver to bond a fluoroquinolone antibiotic to Dacron grafts was described. Silver was noted to provide two distinct advantages: it has inherent antibacterial activity, and it provides an ionic silver-antibiotic complex that is stable for weeks rather than hours or days. Subsequently Modak et al from the same group demonstrated in experiments with oxacillin, a fluoroquinolone and an aminoglycoside that vascular grafts bonded with silver-antibiotic have higher antibacterial activity than those bonded with either agent alone.[18] Silver was found to both increase the uptake and prolong the release of antibiotic. In 1988 these investigators reported the incorporation of silver with oxacillin or amikacin into PTFE grafts using an organic solvent.[19] PTFE was chosen as an early loss of silver-antibiotics was noted in in vivo experiments with Dacron grafts, due to brisk bleeding through the interstices on implantation. Prostheses were implanted in canine aortas and were found to retain 20% of original activity at one week. Grafts infected at operation with *S. aureus* were cultured after one week; antibiotic-impregnated prostheses grew 170-200 colonies versus 1.3 million colonies in controls.

Penicillin-bonded vascular grafts have thus been proven to be superior to untreated and penicillin-soaked grafts in animal models of intraoperative graft infection, without evidence of deleterious consequences. They also appear to be effective in an animal model of established graft infection. Graft explantation in these studies, however, has generally been at three weeks or less following surgery, and it is unclear what long-term protection they will afford. The Greco group describes similar results in grafts explanted at six weeks and three months, yet graft infections may appear at much more remote times. A multicenter clinical trial to test the efficacy of penicillin-bonded vascular grafts in the prevention of graft infections, initiated by Greco and colleagues, is currently underway.

CEPHALOSPORINS

The cephalosporins are a second family of ß-lactam antibiotics. These agents contain a six-membered dihhydrothiazine ring, as opposed to the five-membered thiazolidine ring of the penicillins. (Fig. 2) This structural difference makes the cephalosporins relatively resistant to ß-lactamase. Most cephalosporins in clinical use are semisynthetic derivatives of cephalosporin C, first isolated from the fungus *Cephalosporium acremonium* in 1948. Modifications of the ß-lactam ring side chain alter antibacterial activity, while alterations in the dihydrothiazine ring side chain affect pharmacokinetic properties. The mechanism of action of the cephalosporins is the inhibition of bacterial cell wall synthesis, in essentially the same manner as the penicillins, and thus the mechanisms of bacterial resistance are similar as well. As with the penicillins, absorption, metabolism and excretion vary according to the nature of side chain molecules.

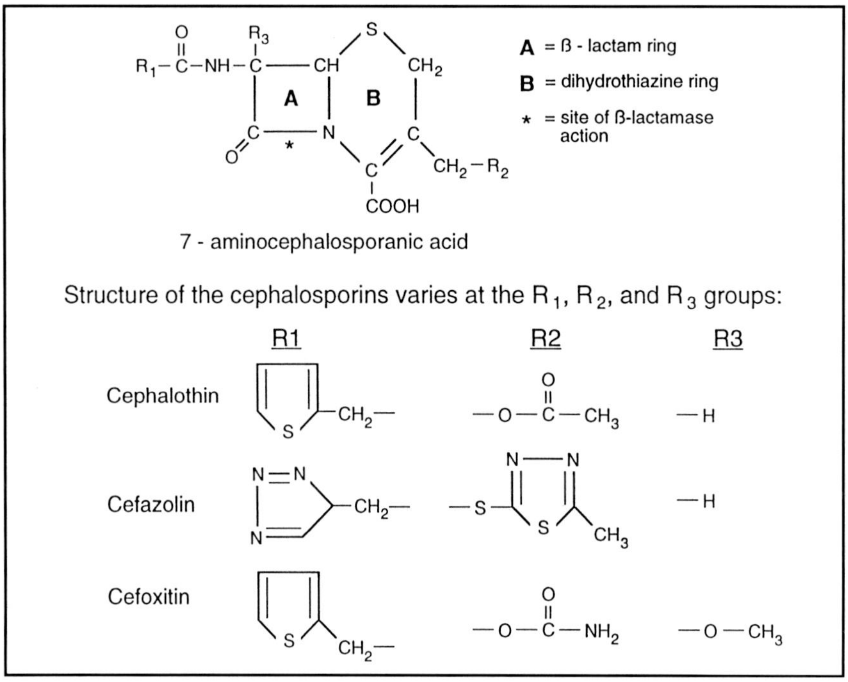

7 - aminocephalosporanic acid

Structure of the cephalosporins varies at the R_1, R_2, and R_3 groups:

Fig. 2. CEPHALOSPORINS

Cephalosporins are grouped according to their antibacterial spectrum into generations. First-generation cephalosporins such as cefazolin and cephalothin are highly active against gram-positive cocci, with the notable exceptions of enterococci, methicillin-resistant *S. aureus* and many strains of *S. epidermidis*. Gram-negative coverage is limited to *E. coli, K. pneumoniae, Pr. mirabilis* and Salmonella and Shigella spp. Anaerobes exclusive of the *B. fragilis* group are included as well. The second-generation cephalosporins such as cefoxitin, cefonocid and cefotetan have improved ß-lactamase stability and are active against a wider range of gram-negative organisms. Anaerobic coverage is extended to include *B. fragilis*. The third generation cephalosporins are highly resistant to ß-lactamase and have high activity against a still wider range of gram-negatives, at lower serum concentrations. They are significantly less active, however, against gram-positive organisms. These include cefotaxime, ceftizoxime and ceftriaxone. A subgroup of the third generation agents are highly active against *Pseudomonas aeruginosa*, including ceftazidine and cefoperazone.

Adverse reactions most commonly consist of delayed hypersensitivity reactions such as rash, fever and eosinophilia. Less common are immediate reactions such as urticaria, bronchospasm and anaphylaxis.

Cross-sensitivity with the penicillins is low despite their similar structure, and patients with penicillin allergy have a less than 5% chance of having the same reaction to a cephalosporin.

CLINICAL AND EXPERIMENTAL USE

The ideal prophylactic antibiotic for surgical procedures should be highly active against the most common pathogens causing postoperative infections, adequately concentrated in serum and at the site of surgery, present in such concentrations throughout the surgical procedure, nontoxic to the patient and of cost reasonable to justify its routine use. For these reasons the cephalosporins have become the antibiotics of choice for the prophylaxis of most vascular surgery procedures. Over 20 years ago it was demonstrated experimentally that cephalosporins are effective in preventing or reducing graft infection in a model of intraoperative bacteremic contamination[20] and a model of local wound contamination.[21] A number of large clinical series have since demonstrated that cephalosporins are vastly superior to placebo[22,23,24] and equal in efficacy to penicillins[6,5] in the prevention of postoperative graft infections. The first generation agents are the cephalosporins most frequently used as their antibacterial spectrum includes three of the most common pathogens involved in vascular graft infections: *S. epidermidis*, *S. aureus* and *E. coli*. Because it has the longest half-life of the first-generation cephalosporins, cefazolin has become the most popular. Resistance to the first-generation cephalosporins among gram-positive organisms, however, is on the rise.

One of the first studies involving the treatment of vascular graft material with antibiotics prior to implantation involved the first-generation cephalosporin Keflin (cefazolin). In 1970 Richardson et al reported that Dacron graft material soaked in cefazolin was infection-resistant compared to saline-soaked controls.[25] Pieces of graft were implanted in subcutaneous pouches in guinea pigs which had been contaminated with *S. aureus* or *E. coli*, removed at eight days and cultured. Although the antibiotics were not bonded to the graft, and the model did not represent an actual vascular surgical procedure. The results did suggest that antibiotics concentrated at the site of surgery could be effective in limiting the deleterious consequences of intraoperative graft contamination.

Despite the fact that they have become the agents of choice for perioperative prophylaxis in vascular surgery, there are surprisingly few reports in the recent literature of the experimental bonding of cephalosporin antibiotics to vascular graft materials. Greco and colleagues have reported the experimental bonding of the second-generation cepha-losporin cefoxitin to PTFE graft material using the organic solvent TDMAC.[26] The cephalosporins, like the penicillins, are anionic molecules which may be bonded to grafts in the same manner as penicillins, using cationic surfactants. In vitro experiments by this group demonstrated that grafts so-treated inhibited the growth of *S. aureus* even after thorough washing and that binding was greater and elution slower with TDMAC than with benzylalkonium. When implanted into rat muscle pouches for ten days, a much higher concentration of antibiotic remained in the TDMAC-bonded group than in antibiotic-soaked controls. TDMAC-bonded grafts were also able to absorb significantly greater amounts of cefoxitin than controls when the antibiotic was administered intravenously or as a local irrigant. In subsequent experiments, however, the group found TDMAC to be significantly more thrombogenic than benzylalkonium.[15]

In 1986 Sobinsky and Flanagan reported that PTFE grafts bonded with cefoxitin by glycosaminoglycan-keratin were successful in preventing infection in a canine model of intraoperative graft contamination.[27] Only 1/10 cefoxitin-treated carotid artery grafts contaminated at implantation with ten million *S. aureus* were infected at explantation, versus 10/10 untreated control grafts. Grafts were harvested at intervals between 1 and 28 days following surgery and no antibiotic could be detected in any grafts after ten days, suggesting that grafts so-treated would initially be infection-resistant but vulnerable to later bacteremic contamination.

AMINOGLYCOSIDES

The aminoglycosides are a group of bactericidal antibiotics which are fermentation products of microorganisms belonging to the genuses Streptomyces and Micronospora. Following the isolation of penicillin from the penicillium mold, a variety of soil actinomycetes were studied to determine if they also produced antimicrobial substances. The first, streptomycin became available for clinical use in 1944, but the rapid development of resistance limited its utility. Since that time over 100 of these agents have been developed, both naturally-occurring aminoglycosides and synthetically altered derivatives. Aminoglycoside antibiotics in common clinical use today include gentamicin and netilmicin, both Micronospora derivatives; tobramycin and neomycin, Streptomyces derivatives; and amikacin, a semisynthetic derivative of kanamycin. (Fig. 3)

The aminoglycosides have rapid bactericidal activity against aerobic gram-negative bacilli and are thus invaluable in the treatment of serious gram-negative infections. They exhibit synergystic activity when administered with ß-lactam antibiotics. Their usefulness against gram-positive organisms is limited. Most streptococci are resistant, and while staphylococci are usually susceptible, plasmid-mediated resistance is becoming widespread in *S. aureus* and *S. epidermidis.*[28,29] They are useful in enterococcal infections only when combined with ß-lactams.[30,31] Anaerobic organisms are naturally resistant as the transport of aminoglycosides into bacterial cells is an energy-dependent, oxygen-requiring process.[32]

The antibacterial action of the aminoglycosides is due to their ability to inhibit protein synthesis and to alter mRNA translation at the ribosome.[33] While most agents which interfere with protein synthesis are bacteriostatic, the aminoglycosides are rapidly bactericidal. It is not yet clear whether the known mechanisms of action adequately explain their rapidity of action.[28] The intracellular targets are the 30S and 50S ribosomes, where they bind and interfere with the initiation of protein synthesis.[34] It also appears that they can cause misreading of mRNA, resulting in the addition of incorrect amino acids into growing peptide chains.[35] Their synergism with the ß-lactams, which impair bacterial cell wall synthesis, results from increased intracellular uptake of aminoglycosides as the bacterial cell wall loses its integrity.[36]

Bacterial resistance is largely due to inactivation of aminoglycosides by plasmid-encoded enzymes. Most of these enzymes alter hydroxyl or amino residues by acetylation, phosphorylation or adenylation. Many semi-synthetic aminoglycosides such as amikacin have been designed so that large side-chain structures protect the antibiotic from these reactions.[30]

The aminoglycosides are water-soluble and strongly cationic. They are not well-absorbed when administered orally. Intramuscular injec-

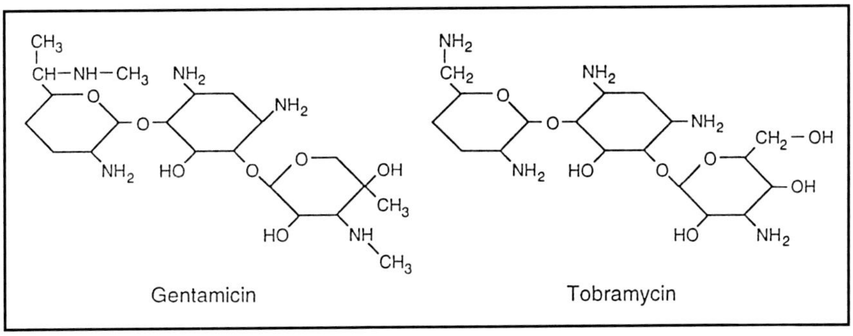

Fig. 3. AMINOGLYCOSIDES

tion produces serum levels similar to intravenous infusion over 30 to 60 minutes. Their polar nature results in negligible intracellular uptake and a volume of distribution approximately equivalent to the extracellular fluid.[37] Poor uptake by cells results in low concentrations in tissue and secretions.[28] The exceptions are the renal medulla and the fluid of the inner ear, accounting for the nephrotoxicity and ototoxicity of these agents.[38] Aminoglycosides are rapidly excreted in unchanged form by glomerular filtration. As the above-mentioned toxicities are related to the serum concentration, it is crucial to alter the dosing of patients with renal insufficiency according to the creatinine clearance. Other reported adverse effects, such as acute neuromuscular blockade and peripheral neuritis, are quite uncommon. Allergic reactions are unusual.

CLINICAL AND EXPERIMENTAL USE

The aminoglycosides have not been widely used clinically as prophylactic agents in vascular surgery, as gram-positive coverage is inconsistent. Plasmid-mediated aminoglycoside resistance in staphylococci is increasing worldwide, and the rapid emergence of mutational resistance during aminoglycoside therapy is well-known. As well, there is a significant population of vascular surgery patients that have underlying renal insufficiency for whom aminoglycosides are, perhaps, a less than ideal choice. They are extremely useful in the treatment of serious gram-negative infections, however, especially in light of their synergystic activity with ß-lactam antibiotics. While the majority of vascular graft infections are due to gram-positive organisms, up to one-half of abdominal graft infections involve gram-negative bacilli.

Moore and colleagues were the first to report experimental results with aminoglycoside-bonded vascular grafts.[39] In a canine model of immediate postoperative bacteremic aortic graft contamination with *S. aureus*, velour prostheses with collagen-bound amikacin were found to significantly reduce the incidence of graft infection compared to grafts containing collagen alone. Animals received an intravenous infusion of ten million *S. aureus* after wound closure and grafts were explanted at three weeks. Only 1/12 experimental grafts were infected compared to 13/13 controls. When residual antibiotic activity was assessed, only 1/12 experimental grafts retained bacterial inhibition, indicating that the protective effect did not extend beyond the immediate postoperative period. In 1989 Shenk et al reported the use of cyanoacrylate with tobramycin powder to form an "antibiotic glue," which was applied to PTFE aortic grafts following implantation in a canine model of intraoperative graft contamination.[40] Grafts were immersed in solutions of 30 million organisms each of *E. coli* and *S. aureus* prior to placement. Upon reoperation at three days, 11/11 untreated controls were culture-positive and 7/11 had pseudoaneurysms, versus none of four treated animals. The ten surviving control animals underwent replacement of the infected graft, and five of these were treated at surgery with the tobramycin glue. On explantation at two weeks graft cultures were positive in all of the controls and negative in all of the treated grafts. This group has also reported the treatment of PTFE grafts in the same model with a fibrin glue-tobramycin suspension which was made by combining cryoprecipitate, thrombin, aminocaproic acid and the antibiotic. Graft infection was reduced and survival improved in animals treated with this suspension, compared to those which were untreated or treated with fibrin glue alone. Cultures of antibiotic-treated grafts, however, remained positive for *S. aureus* in 3/4 and for *E. coli* and Pseudomonas in 1/4 when explanted at 17 days.

New aminoglycosides with increased gram-positive activity are currently in development. Haverich and colleagues have reported the topical application of the gentamicin derivative EMD 46/217, a long-acting and poorly soluble aminoglycoside with a spectrum of activity that includes *S. aureus* and *S. epidermidis,* to Dacron prosthetic material.[41] In vitro elution expeiments revealed antibiotic release for three weeks when applied to Dacron using a fibrin sealant. Treated graft rings were then contaminated with *S. aureus* and implanted intraluminally in porcine aortas on a steel mounting device. Upon removal at one week, significant amounts of EMD 46/217 were retained in the fibrin-treated grafts versus none in those treated with antibiotic alone. In this study, 5/10 experimental grafts were sterile at explantation, versus only 1/10 antibiotic-soaked grafts and none of the controls.

FLUOROQUINOLONES

The fluoroquinolones are relatively new class of antibiotics, available for clinical use in the United States for only a few years. Originally developed as orally administered, broad-spectrum agents, fluoroquinolones are now becoming available in injectable form. These drugs exhibit great activity against most aerobic and facultative gram-negative organisms, with only moderate activity against gram-positive organisms. However, MICs are 1 mg/ml or less for many staphylococci and streptococci, including MRSA. Activity against anaerobes is relatively

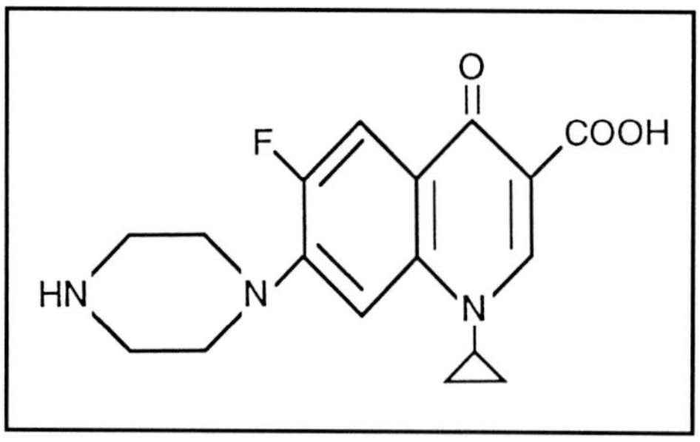

Fig. 4. CIPRLOXACIN

poor. Fluoroquinolones are also active against mycobacteria, chlamydia and rickettsia. Several new fluoroquinolones are in development which have greatly improved anti-gram-positive activity.[42] (Fig. 4)

Quinolone antibiotics are synthetic agents, the oldest of which is nalidixic acid. Those in current clinical use are fluorinated 4-quinolones, which are much less prone to the development of bacterial resistance than their precursors. The mechanism of action of this class of bactericidal antibiotics has yet to be completely elucidated. It has been established, however, that the fluoroquinolones interfere with the activity of DNA gyrase, an enzyme essential for DNA synthesis.[43,44] DNA gyrase is a tetramer of two A and two B subunits; the A subunit is the target structure.[45] Quinolones appear to bind directly to DNA rather than the enzyme itself, and then form a quinolone-DNA-gyrase complex which results in a decrease in DNA synthesis.[46] In vitro studies have demonstrated that there is a close but not absolute relationship between antigyrase activity and antibacterial potency. While this may be explained in part by varying bacterial penetration between quinolones, it has been suggested that there may be other as yet unknown intracellular targets.

Fluoroquinolone antibiotics exhibit a number of favorable pharmacokinetic properties which are distinctly different from the ß-lactams and aminoglycosides. They have a long half-life, a wide volume of distribution, minimal binding to serum protein and two-pathway elimination kinetics.[47] They are able to achieve tissue-to-serum ratios in excess of 2:1, as compared to the ß-lactams which rarely exhibit tissue to serum levels greater than 0.4:1.[48,49] This is possible because fluoroquinolones freely penetrate cell membranes and ionically bind to intracellular structures. Additionally, infected sites have higher fluoroquinolone tissue-to-serum ratios than uninfected tissues of the same type, potentially a result of binding to accumulating leukocytes.[47,50]

Fluoroquinolones are metabolized in the liver to less active piperazine and inactive glucuronide derivatives. Excretion is by biliary or renal routes or both. Ciprofloxacin, for example, is excreted by both routes, and therefore does not accumulate excessively in patients with liver disease or in those with renal insufficiency.[51]

Resistance to the fluoroquinolones appears to be mediated by mutations in the chromosomal genes for DNA gyrase and for membrane permeability proteins called porins.[44,52] Clinically these mechanisms of resistance develop slowly. Because of their unique mechanism of action, cross-resistance with other antibiotics is limited. There has been no reported evidence of plasmid-mediated resistance.[53]

CLINICAL AND EXPERIMENTAL USE

Ciprofloxacin (Fig. 4) was the first of the fluoroquinolones to be marketed in the U.S. Initially available only for oral administration, these broad-spectrum agents have been used widely in respiratory, urinary tract, bone and joint and other infections. Recently an injectable form of ciprofloxacin has become available for clinical use. The broad antibacterial spectrum, excellent tissue penetration and low toxicity of the fluoroquinolones make them potentially ideal agents for the prophylaxis of surgical infections. Limited data is available concerning the use of fluoroquinolones for this indication, however there are reports of efficacy equal or superior to that of cephalosporin antibiotics in the prophylaxis of colorectal,[54,55] biliary[56,57] and urologic surgery.[58,59,60] Auger et al have reported a randomized study of pefloxacin, a nalidixic acid analogue and cefazolin in patients undergoing cardiac surgery.[61] Of 111 patients, 14 receiving perifloxacin developed bacterial colonization at culture sites versus 11 in the cefazolin group. One patient who received cefazolin developed mediastinitis from a cefazolin-resistant strain of *S. epidermidis.* As yet there are no published clinical trials of a fluoroqinolone versus a cephalosporin in the prophylaxis of peripheral vascular surgery procedures.

White and colleagues reported the soaking of knitted Dacron grafts in silver-pefloxacin in 1984.[17] Using radiolabelled silver complexes, it was demonstrated that significant antibacterial activity remained in these grafts after 19 days of washing. When tested in a canine model of intraoperative hematogenous aortic graft contamination with *S. aureus,* 1/6 silver-pefloxacin-treated grafts were found to have positive cultures on explantation at three weeks, versus 9/11 controls. In 1987 this group reported in vitro and in vivo experiments in which norfloxacin and pefloxacin, as well as oxacillin and sulfadiazine, were bonded to PTFE graft material with and without silver.[18] Grafts bonded with silver demonstrated increased uptake and prolonged release of antibiotic.

In 1991 Kinney and colleagues reported an in vivo elution experiment in which ciprofloxacin-bonded PTFE grafts were implanted in canine carotid and femoral arteries, and then explanted at various intervals to determine antibacterial potency.[62] Grafts bonded with ciprofloxacin and silver sustained the highest level of antibiotic potency at 14 days, with an antibiotic concentration well in excess of the MIC for *S. epidermidis*. To date there are no reports of fluoroquinolone-treated grafts in animal models of established graft infection. Kinney et al postulate that an antibiotic-bonded graft with sustained release might be useful in the replacement of infected grafts, and they are currently studying the utility of such grafts versus systemic antibiotics and graft replacement alone in a model of established graft infection.

RIFAMPIN

The rifamycins are a group of complex, macrocyclic antibiotics produced by *Streptomyces mediterranei*. Rifampin is a semisynthetic, broad-spectrum antibiotic derivative of rifamycin B, and it is the only antibiotic of this class in wide clinical use. It is highly active against most gram-positive bacteria. Bactericidal concentrations against *Staphylococcus aureus* and coagulase-negative staphylococcus are as low as 0.005 mg/ml.[63] It is also highly active against M. tuberculosis and most nontuberculous mycobacteria. Activity against the gram-negatives is variable. (Fig. 5)

Rifampin is bactericidal for intra- and extracellular organisms. It suppresses the initiation of RNA synthesis by binding to and inhibiting DNA-dependent RNA polymerase. The counterpart of this enzyme in mammalian cell nuclei is insensitive to rifampin. The mammalian

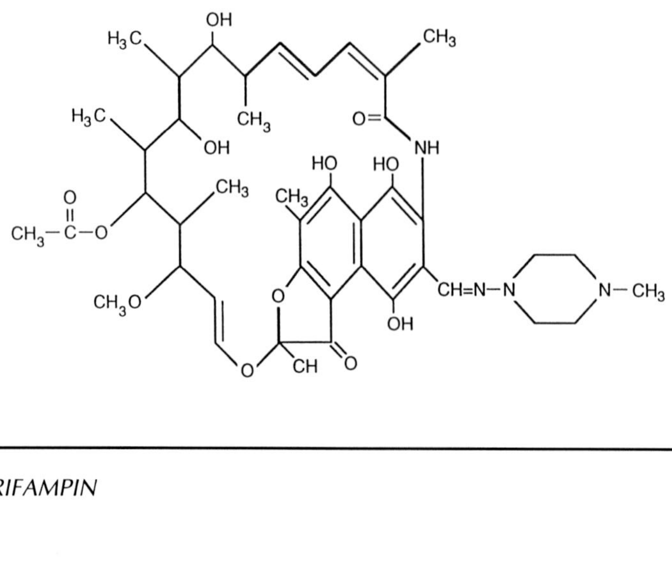

Fig. 5. RIFAMPIN

mitochondrial RNA polymerase is sensitive, but it appears that rifampin is not able to cross the mitochondrial membrane in quantities sufficient to inhibit RNA synthesis.[64,65] Like the aminoglycosides, synergism with drugs that inhibit cell wall synthesis has been demonstrated.[66] Resistance to rifampin develops rapidly in vitro and in vivo when the drug is used alone. This occurs as a one-step mutation (in a single generation) and results in a change in the structure of RNA polymerase which decreases the ability of rifampin to bind to it. This phenomenon has been observed in most bacteria sensitive to rifampin, including the mycobacteria, gram-positive cocci and gram-negative rods.[65] rifampin must not be administered alone, therefore, in the treatment of active infections. Resistant strains may emerge despite multiagent therapy, as rifampin resistance has been reported in *S. aureus* and *S. epidermidis* during rifampin/vancomycin combination therapy.[67,68] A form of natural resistance has also been suggested which relates to variability in permeability barriers.[69]

Rifampin is usually administered orally, although an IV preparation is available for patients unable to take oral medications. It is excreted in the bile both unchanged and in a deacetlylated, but active, form. It undergoes enterohepatic recirculation, but the metabolized form is poorly reabsorbed. High levels of rifampin may accumulate in patients with liver disease or biliary obstruction. Urinary excretion is related to serum levels and accumulation docs not occur in patients with renal insufficiency.[65]

Tissue penetration of rifampin is excellent, with concentrations in some viscera exceeding serum levels. It possesses the unusual property among antibiotics of being lipid-soluble, and is therefore able to freely penetrate the cell membrane and attack intracellular organisms. It has been suggested that this may be of value in the eradication of intracellular staphylococci which are present in leukocyte collections.[68]

Rifampin is usually well-tolerated, with adverse reactions reported in 5% or less of patients. Most common are rash, fever and gastrointestinal complaints. Serious reactions, such as hepatitis and nephritis, are rare. Rifampin is a potent inducer of hepatic microsomal enzymes and thus causes accelerated metabolism of a number of drugs.

CLINICAL AND EXPERIMENTAL USE

While rifampin is not in common clinical use in vascular surgery prophylaxis, its extremely high anti-staphylococcal activity has stimulated a great deal of investigational interest in recent years. Its high level of activity against *S. epidermidis* and *S. aureus* at MICs generally less than 0.008 mg/ml make it a potentially ideal antibiotic for this indication. Rutledge et al reported in 1982 that a preoperative intramuscular injection of rifampin was superior to cefazolin administered in the same fashion in a canine model of intraoperative graft infection.[70] Following the placement of PTFE carotid arterial grafts, 1000 *S. aureus* organisms sensitive to both antibiotics were injected over the grafts. The grafts were removed after five days and cultured. Only 2/12 grafts were infected in the rifampin-treated group, compared to 7/12 in the cefazolin-treated group and 7/7 untreated controls.

Wakefield and colleagues hypothesized that antibiotics such as rifampin which are concentrated in leukocytes might be highly effective in treating established graft infections.[71] This group tested intravenous rifampin and clindamycin versus cefazolin in a canine model of intraoperative aortic graft contamination. Dacron aortic grafts were infected with 100 million *S. aureus* immediately after implantation; at three months following surgery a four week course of antibiotic therapy was initiated after which grafts were removed for quantitative bacteriologic study. 7/7 grafts treated with rifampin and clindamycin were sterile, compared to 5/7 cefazolin-treated grafts. Of three untreated control grafts, one had thrombosed and two were contaminated. Although the rifampin/clindamycin group fared better than the cefazolin group, the difference was not statistically significant. It is not possible to discern the individual effect of rifampin versus that of clindamycin from this experiment.

The vast majority of laboratory investigation into the use of rifampin as a prophylactic agent in vascular surgery, however, has focused on the incorporation of rifampin into graft materials to produce an infection-resistant vascular prosthesis. As it has the ability to inhibit the growth of bacteria at such minute concentrations, a rifampin-bonded vascular graft might retain antibacterial activity for much longer periods of time than grafts bonded with antibiotics which have higher MICs. Additionally, its relative insolubility in water results in a much slower elution from graft materials when passively absorbed. Powell and colleagues, from the same group as Rutledge, described the passive incorporation of rifampin into Dacron grafts by adding it to the blood used for preclotting.[72] Grafts were implanted in canine aortas, harvested at varying intervals and tested for antibiotic activity. Treated grafts retained 94% of their original ability to inhibit the growth of *S. aureus* on agar plates at 6 hours and 91% at 24 hours. These passively treated grafts were then tested in a canine model of hematogenous perioperative aortic graft contamination.[73] Three groups of five animals had Dacron grafts preclotted with blood containing rifampin, cefazolin or saline. An intravenous infusion of ten million *S. aureus* known to be sensitive to both antibiotics was administered in the perioperative period. On explantation at three weeks, 0/5 rifampin-treated grafts had clinical or culture evidence of infection, versus 5/5 cefazolin-treated grafts and 3/5 controls. No grafts were found to possess residual antibiotic activity at the end of the experiment by zone of inhibition assays, indicating that passive incorporation of rifampin would be unlikely to afford long-term protection.

Other groups have reported the use of protein sealants to bond rifampin to graft material. Strachan et al describe the ionic bonding of rifampin to carboxyl moieties on gelatin-sealed Dacron.[74] Grafts treated in this manner have been implanted in four patients at high risk of postoperative infection. Avramovic and Fletcher have also reported in vitro and in vivo success with this passive method of rifampin bonding.[75,76] In an ovine model of intraoperative local contamination of carotid artery grafts, rifampin-treated grafts were relatively infection-resistant with only 2/10 infected at three weeks versus 6/8 controls.

Chervu and colleagues have attempted to circumvent the problem of rapid elution of rifampin by using minimally cross-linked type I collagen to bind antibiotics to Dacron graft material. In an in vitro elution experiment this group demonstrated that collagen-bonded rifampin grafts had an average duration of activity against *S. aureus* of over 22 days, compared to 2 days or less for grafts bonded with amikacin or chloramphenicol in the same manner.[77] Grafts preclotted with rifampin-containing blood had an average duration of antibiotic activity of less than six days. Having shown that collagen bonding can provide a sustained-release system for rifampin, the investigators then tested these grafts in a canine model of postoperative hematogenous graft infection.[78] Four groups of six dogs, each with its own group of control grafts treated with collagen alone, had aortic grafts implanted which were contaminated hematogenously with 120 million *S. aureus* at 2, 7, 10 or 12 days following surgery. Grafts were harvested three weeks after contamination. Of those contaminated at two and seven days, none of the experimental grafts were infected, versus 4/6 and 5/6 of their controls, respectively. In the ten day group 1/6 experimental grafts and only 2/6 controls were infected; in the 12 day group 2/6 experimental grafts and 1/6 controls were infected. The investigators conclude that grafts treated in this manner are infection-resistant for seven days following implantation and suggest that accelerated healing of the collagen graft surface may protect against delayed bacterial seeding.

These investigators have also tested collagen-bonded rifampin grafts in a model of established graft infection.[79] Grafts were implanted in canine infrarenal aortas and contaminated with 100 S. *aureus* prior to wound closure. This small inoculum of bacteria produced a clinical infection in 100% of animals. One week following the initial surgery the grafts were removed, the graft bed debrided and either a new rifampin-impregnated graft (n=47) or an untreated control graft (n=36) was implanted at the same site. Animals were further randomized to receive no supplemental antibiotics or one of three antibiotic protocols: perioperative cefazolin only, cefazolin for one week or cefazolin for two weeks. Among control grafts, infection rates were 100%, 87.5%, 100% and 80%, respectively. Among the rifampin-bonded grafts, infection rates were 50%, 50%, 20% and 20%, respectively. Rifampin-bonded Dacron prostheses were thus able to reduce the incidence of subsequent bacterial growth in a grossly infected arterial bed.

CONCLUSIONS

Prophylactic antibiotics clearly reduce the incidence of postoperative graft infection in vascular surgery. Because of their favorable pharmacologic and pharmacokinetic properties, the cephalosporins are currently the antibiotic of choice for this indication. There is evidence that fluoroquinolones may be as effective and even superior to cephalosporins in a number of settings in surgical prophylaxis, however this has yet to be demonstrated in peripheral vascular surgery where prosthetic graft materials are used.

The desire to concentrate antibiotics at the site of potential infection has logically led to efforts to incorporate antibiotics into vascular prostheses. This method of delivery would also avoid the potential complications and expense of systemic antibiotic administration. The development of antibiotic-treated vascular grafts began over 20 years ago and has involved almost the entire spectrum of antibiotic agents in common clinical use. In recent years it has become one of the most rapidly growing areas of experimental investigation in vascular surgery.

It has become clear that antibiotics must be bonded to graft materials in order to prevent rapid elution and loss of antibacterial activity. The method of bonding employed must be tailored to the chemical nature of individual antibiotic agents. There is experimental evidence that significant antibiotic activity may be retained in some grafts in vitro for up to three weeks and in vivo for over one week. It may also be possible to "recharge" some grafts postoperatively by systemic antibiotic administration.

The questions of which antibiotic agent is most appropriate and what duration of antibiotic activity is necessary have not yet been answered. There is essentially only anecdotal clinical experience to date with antibiotic-treated vascular prostheses. The safety and efficacy of these grafts remain to be proven in prospective, randomized clinical trials. Their remarkable success in many highly challenging animal models of graft infection suggests that antibiotic-treated grafts may well change the manner in which vascular surgery patients are managed, in both routine vascular reconstruction and the treatment of infected prostheses.

REFERENCES

1. Greenwood D. Antibiotics of the beta-lactam group. New York: Research Studies Press, 1982:84.
2. Mandell G, Sande M. Penicillins, cephalosporins and other beta-lactam antibiotics. In: Gilman A, Rall T, Nies A, Taylor P, eds. The Pharmacologic Basis of Therapeutics. Elmsford, NY: Pergamon Press, 1990: 1065-1097.
3. Molavi A, LeFrock J. Antistaphylococcal penicillins. In: Ristuccia A, Cunha B, ed. Antimicrobial Therapy. New York: Raven Press, 1984: 183-195.
4. Idsoe O, Guthe T, Willcox R, DeWeck A. Nature and extent of penicillin side-reactions with particular reference to fatalities from anaphylactic shock. Bull WHO 1968; 38: 159-188.
5. Goldstone J, Moore W. Infection in vascular prosthesis. Am J Surg 1974; 128: 225-233.
6. May A, Darling R, Brewster D, Darling C. A comparison of the use of cephalothin and oxacillin in vascular surgery. Arch Surg 1980; 115: 56-59.
7. Henry R, Jagpal R, Greco R. Antibiotic bonding to a polyfluorotetraethylene surface. Assoc Acad Surg 1979; 13: 30-36.
8. Jagpal R, Greco R. Studies on a graphite-benzalkonium-oxacillin surface. Am Surg 1979; 45: 774-779.
9. Henry R, Harvey R, Greco R. Antibiotic bonding to vascular prosthesis. J Thor Cardiovasc Surg 1981; 82: 272-277.
10. Prahlad A, Harvey R, Greco R. Diffusion of antibiotics from a polyfluorotetraethylene-benzalkonium surface. Am Surg 1981; 47: 515-518.
11. Harvey R, Alcid D, Greco R. Antibiotic bonding to polyfluorotetraethylene with tridodecylmethylammonium chloride. Surgery 1982; 92: 504-512.
12. Greco R, Harvey R, Henry R, Prahlad A. Prevention of graft infection by antibiotic bonding. Surg Forum 1980; 31: 29-30.
13. Greco R, Harvey R. The role of antibiotic bonding in the prevention of vascular prosthetic infections. Ann Surg 1982; 195: 168-171.
14. Greco R, Harvey R, Smilow P, Tesoriero J. Prevention of vascular prosthetic infection by a benzalkonium-oxacillin bonded polytetrafluoroethylene graft. Surg Gynecol Obstet 1982; 155: 28-32.
15. Greco R, Trooskin S, Donetz A, Harvey R. The application of antibiotic bonding to the treatment of established vascular prosthetic infection. Arch Surg 1985; 120: 71-

75.

16. Shue W, Worosilo S, Donetz A et al. Prevention of vascular prosthetic unfection with an antibiotic-bonded Dacron graft. J Vasc Surg 1988; 8: 600-605.

17. White J, Benvenisty A, Reemtsma K et al. Simple methods for direct antibiotic protection of synthetic vascular grafts. J Vasc Surg 1984; 1: 372-380.

18. Modak S, Sampath L, Fox C et al. A new method for the direct incorporation of antibiotic in prosthetic vascular grafts. Surg Gynecol Obstet 1987; 164: 143-147.

19. Benvenisty A, Tannembaum G, Ahlnorn T et al. Control of prosthetic bacterial infection: Evaluation of an easily incorporated, tightly bound, silver antibiotic PTFE graft. J Surg Res 1988; 44: 1-7.

20. Moore W, Rosson C, Hall A. Effect of prophylactic antibiotics in preventing bacteremic infection in vascular prostheses. Surgery 1971; 69: 825-828.

21. Lindenauer S, Fry W, Schaub G, Wild D. The use of antibiotics in the prevention of vascular graft infections. Surgery 1967; 62: 487-492.

22. Kaiser A, Clayson K, Mulberin J et al. Antibiotic prophylaxis in vascular surgery. Ann Surg 1978; 188: 283-289.

23. Salzmann G. Perioperative infection prophylaxis in vascular surgery: A randomized prospective study. Thorac Cardiovasc Surg 1983; 31: 239-242.

24. Hasselgren P, Ivarsson L, Risberg B, Seeman T. Effects of prophylactic antibiotics in vascular surgery. Ann Surg 1984; 200: 86-92.

25. Richardson R, Pate J, Wolf R et al. The outcome of antibiotic-soaked arterial grafts in guinea pig wounds contaminated with *E. coli* or *S. aureus.* J Thorac Cardiovasc Surg 1970; 59: 635-637.

26. Greco R, Harvey R. The biochemical bonding of cefoxitin to a microporous polytetrafluoroethylene surface. J Surg Res 1984; 36: 237-243.

27. Sobinsky K, Flanigan D. Antibiotic binding to polytetrafluoroethylene via glucosaminoglycan-keratin luminal coating. Surgery 1986; 100: 629-634.

28. Sande M, Mandell G. The Aminoglycosides. In: Gilman A, Rall T, Nies A, Taylor P, ed. The Pharmacologic Basis of Therapeutics. Elmsford, NY: Pergamon Press, 1990: 1098-1116.

29. Mitsuhashi S, Kawabe H. Aminoglycoside antibiotic resistance in bacteria. In: Whelton A, Neu H, ed. The Aminoglycosides: Microbiology, Clinical Use and Toxicology. New York: Marcel Dekker, 1982: 97-122.

30. Ristuccia A. Aminoglycosides. In: Ristuccia A, Cunha B, ed. Antimicrobial Therapy. New York: Raven Press, 1984: 305-328.

31. Moellering RJ, Wennersten C, Weinberg A. Studies on antibiotic synergism against enterococci. I.Bacteriologic studies. J Lab Clin Med 1971; 77: 821-828.

32. Verklin RJ, Mandell G. Alteration of effectiveness of antibiotics by anaerobiasis. J Lab Clin Med 1977; 89: 65-71.

33. Shannon K, Phillips I. Mechanisms of resistance to aminoglycosides in clinical isolates. J Antimicrob Chemother 1982; 9: 91-102.

34. Davies B. The lethal action of aminoglycosides. J Antimicrob Chemother 1988; 22: 1-3.

35. Tai P-C, Wallace B, Davis B. Streptomycin causes misreading of natural messenger by interacting with ribosomes after initiation. Proc Natl Acad Sci USA 1978; 75: 275-279.

36. Moellering RJ. Clinical microbiology and the in vitro activity of aminoglycosides. In: Whelton A, Neu H, ed. The Aminoglycosides. New York: Marcel Dekker, 1982: 65-

95.
37. Barza M, Brown R, D S, Gibaldi M, Weinstein L. Predictability of blood levels of gentamicin in man. J Infect Dis 1975; 132: 165-174.
38. Davies B, Brummett R, Bendrick T, Himes D. Dissociation of maximum concentration of kanamycin in plamsa and perilymph from ototoxic effect. J Antimicrob Chemother 1984; 14: 291-302.
39. Moore W, Chvapil M, Seiffert G, Keown K. Development of an infection-resistant vascular prosthesis. Arch Surg 1981; 116: 1403-1407.
40. Shenk J, Ney A, Tsykayama D et al. Tobramycin-adhesive in preventing and treating PTFE vascular graft infections. J Surg Res 1989; 47: 487-492.
41. Haverich A, Hirt S, Karck M et al. Prevention of graft infection by bonding of gentamicin to Dacron prostheses. J Vasc Surg 1992; 15: 187-193.
42. Espinosa A, Chin N-X, Novelli A, Neu H. Comparative *in vitro* activity of a new fluorinated 4-quinolone, T-3262 (A-60969). Antimicrob Agents Chemother 1988; 32: 663-670.
43. Smith J. The mode of action of 4-quinolones and possible mechanisms of resistance. J Antimicrob Chemother 1986; 18(suppl D): 21-29.
44. Hooper D, Wolfson J, Souza K et al. Genetic and biochemical characterization of norfloxacin resistance in *Escherichia coli*. Antimicrob Agents Chemother 1986; 29: 639-644.
45. Gellert M, Mizuuchi K, O'Dea M. DNA gyrase: an enzyme that introduces superhelical turns into DNA. Proc Natl Acad Sci USA 1976; 73: 3872-3876.
46. Tabary X, Moraeu N, Dureuil C, LeGoffic F. Effect of DNA gyrase inhibitors perfloxacin, five other quinolones, novobiocin and clorobiocin on *Escheriichia coli* topoisomerase I. Antimicrob Agents Chemother 1987; 31: 1925-1928.
47. Schentag J, Nix D. Pharmacokinetics and tissue penetration of the fluoroquinolones. In: Sanders WJ, Sanders C, ed. Fluoroquinolones in the treatment of infectious diseases. Glenview, IL: Physicians and Scientists Publishing, 1990: 29-44.
48. Neuman M. Clinical pharmacokinetics of the newer antimicrobial 4-quinolones. Clin Pharmacokinetics 1988; 14: 96-121.
49. Schentag J, Gengo F. Principles of antibiotic tissue penetration and guidelines for pharmacokinetic analysis. Med Clin N Am 1982; 66: 39-49.
50. Garlando F, Reitiker S, Tauber M et al. Single-dose ciprofloxacin at 100 versus 250 mg for treatment of uncomplicated urinary tract infections in women. Antimicrob Agents Chemother 1987; 31: 354-356.
51. Nix D, Schentag J. The quinolones: An overview and comparative appraisal of their pharmacokinetics and pharmacodynamics. J Clin Pharmacol 1988; 28: 169-172.
52. Hirai K, Aoyoma H, Suzue S et al. Isolation and characterization of norfloxacin-resistant mutants of *Escherichia coli* K-12. Animicrob Agents Chemother 1986; 30: 248-253.
53. Sanders C. Microbiology of Fluoroquinolones. In: Sanders WJ, Sanders C, ed. Fluoroquinolones in the treatment of infectious diseases. Glenview, IL: Physicians and Scientists Publishing Company, 1990: 1-27.
54. Offer C, Weuta H, Bodner E. Efficacy of perioperative prophylaxis with ciprofloxacin of cefazolin in colorectal surgery. Infection 1988; 16(suppl 1): S46-S47.
55. Cooreman F, Ghyselen J, Penninckx F. Pefloxacin versus cefuroxime for prophylaxis of infections after elective colorectal surgery. Rev Infect Dis 1989; 11(suppl 5): S1301.
56. Kujath P. Brief report: Antibiotic prophylaxis in biliary tract surgery: Ciprofloxacin

versus ceftriaxone. Am J Med 1989; 87(suppl 5A): 255S-257S.

57. Cooreman F. Pefloxacin versus cefazolin as single-dose prophylaxis in elective biliary tract surgery. Rev Infect Dis 1989; 11(suppl 5): S1300.

58. Gombert M, DuBouchet L, Aulicino T et al. Brief report: Intravenous ciprofloxacin versus cefotaxime prophylaxis during transurethral surgery. Am J Med 1989; 87(suppl 5A): 250S-251S.

59. Cox C. Comparison of intravenous ciprofloxacin and intravenous cefotaxime for antimicrobial prophylaxis in transurethral surgery. Am J Med 1989; 87(suppl 5A): 252S-254S.

60. Christensen M, Nielsen K, Knes J, Madsen P. Brief report: Single-dose preoperative prophylaxis in transurethral surgery - Ciprofloxacin versus cefotaxime. Am J Med 1989; 87(suppl 5A): 258S-260S.

61. Auger P, Leclerc Y, Pelletier L et al. Efficacy and safety of pefloxacin versus cefazolin as prophylaxis in elective cardiovascular surgery. Rev Infect Dis 1989; 11(suppl 5): S1302-S1303.

62. Kinney E, Bandyk D, Seabrook G et al. Antibiotic-bonded PTFE vascular grafts: The effect of silver antibiotic on bioactivity following implantation. J Surg Res 1991; 50: 430-435.

63. Farr B, Mandell G. Rifampin. Med Clin N Am 1982; 66: 157-168.

64. Mandell G, Sande M. Drugs used in the chemotherapy of tuberculosis and leprosy. In: Gilman A, Rall T, Nies A, Taylor P, ed. The Pharmacological Basis of Therapeutics. Elmsford, NY: Pergamon Press, 1990: 1146-1164.

65. Kucers A, Bennett N. Rifampicin. In: Kucers A, Bennett N, ed. The Use of Antibiotics. Philadelphia: J. P. Lippincott Co., 1987: 914-970.

66. Zinner S, Lagast H, Klastersky J. Antistaphylococcal activity of rifampin with other antibiotics. J Infect Dis 1981; 144: 365-375.

67. Acar R, Goldstein F, Duval J. Use of rifampin for the treatment of serious stpahylococcal and Gram-negative bacillary infections. Rev Infect Dis 1983; 5 (Suppl. 3): S502-S506.

68. Simon G, Smith R, Sande M. Emergence of rifampin-resistant strains of Staphylococcus aureus during combination therapy with vancomycin and rifampin: a report of two cases. Rev Infect Dis 1983; 5 (Suppl. 3): S507-S514.

69. Hui J, Gordon N, Kajioka R. Permeability barrier to rifampicin in mycobacteria. Antimicrob Ag Chemother 1977; 11: 773-779.

70. Rutledge R, Baker V, Shertz R, Johnson G. Rifampin and cefazolin as prophylactic agents. Arch Surg 1982; 117: 1164-1165.

71. Wakefield T, Schaberg D, Pierson C et al. Treatment of established prosthetic vascular graft infection with antibiotics preferentially concentrated in leucocytes. Surgery 1987; 102: 8-14.

72. Powell T, Burnham S, Johnson G Jr. A passive system using rifampin to create an infection-resistant vascular prosthesis. Surgery 1983; 94: 765-769.

73. McDougal E, Burnham S, Johnson G J. Rifampin protection against experimental graft sepsis. J Vasc Surg 1986; 4: 5-7.

74. Strachan C, Newsom S, Ashton T. The clinical use of an antibiotic-bonded graft. Eur J Vasc Surg 1991; 5: 627-632.

75. Avramovic J, Fletcher J. Rifampicin impregnation of a protein-sealed Dacron graft: An infection resistant prosthetic vascular graft. Aust NZ J Surg 1991; 61: 436-440.

76. Avramovic J, Fletcher J. Prevention of prosthetic vascular graft infection by rifampicin impregnation of a protein-sealed Dacron graft in combination with parenteral cephalosporin. J Cardiovasc Surg 1991; 33: 70-74.
77. Chervu A, Moore W, Chvapil M, Henderson T. Efficacy and duration of antistaphylococcal activity comparing three antibiotics bonded to Dacron vascualr grafts with a collagen release system. J Vasc Surg 1991; 13: 897-901.
78. Chervu A, Moore W, Gelabert H et al. Prevention of graft infection by use of prosthesis bonded with a rifampin/collagen release system. J Vasc Surg 1991; 14(4): 521-525.
79. Chervu A, Moore W, Gelabert H et al. J Vasc Surg 1992 (in press).

CHAPTER 4

GRAFT MATERIALS

George E. Hajjar

HISTORICAL DEVELOPMENT

The first use of a conduit to bridge an arterial defect probably dates back to the 1900s with the experiments of Carrel and Guthrie. They reported the successful experimental transplant of a dog's vena cava into the carotid artery. Other reports appeared at that time describing different arterial repairs in humans utilizing segments of autogenous veins.[1]

ARTERIAL ALLOGRAFTS

In the 1940s and 1950s arterial homografts generated considerable interest. Gross harvested and preserved arterial segments from victims of fatal trauma and used these in the surgical repair of cardiovascular defects.[2] Histological observations revealed that the cellular elements which constituted these grafts were soon lost. Further, the interaction of the host and graft cells could incite an inflammatory response. This led to interest in nonviable arterial homografts.[3] With increasing demand for arterial replacement surgery, the clinical use of nonviable arterial homografts was popularized in the mid-1950s by surgeons such as DeBakey[4] and Szilagyi.[5] Shortly thereafter, complications associated with the use of these grafts were noted.

Graft thrombosis and occlusion were noted in several instances in which progression of the native arterial disease was unlikely.[6] Linton reported a two- to three-year follow-up graft patency rate of only 60%.[7] Late graft degeneration with pseudoaneurysm formation became a recognized sequella. In rare instances, active rejection of the biological graft material was documented. With these new disappointing reports the enthusiasm for denatured biological aortic grafts faded and a quest for a new graft material had begun. An alternate conduit was required.

SYNTHETIC GRAFTS

The modern era of synthetic vascular grafting owes its existence to the efforts of Voorhees and his associates in 1952.[8] While working on an experimental dog model for cardiac valve replacement, they noted that silk sutures became coated with a glistening film free of thrombi. This led to the concept of biocompatibility: that certain materials could be placed within the circulatory system and would not lead to rejection or significant thrombosis. The field was open to the development of synthetic arteries.

Early cylindrical arterial prostheses were fashioned from Vinyon "N" cloth and implanted as replacement segments for dog aortas. Later examination of the harvested prostheses showed that the inner surface became coated with the neointima, which consisted of flattened fibroblasts and collagen fibers. Fibrin plugs formed between the interstices and prevented hemorrhage from the wall of the prosthesis. Shortly thereafter, the first reports of clinical use of synthetic material as arterial replacement started appearing and the search for the ideal synthetic vascular prosthesis had begun.[9] The search evolved through various substances, nylon; Teflon, Orlon and Dacron. In addition to the variety of materials, a variety of graft construction techniques were also being investigated: knitted, woven, crimped and velour; each with its own set of advantages and disadvantages. Their principal disadvantage was their inability to resist infections and their tendency to thrombose. Clearly, the native tissues, even when diseased, often possessed some superior properties.

BIOSYNTHETIC GRAFTS

With the realization that a blood vessel is more than an inert conduit, efforts were directed at developing a graft which would closely mimic the biological properties of arteries. This led to a new generation of synthetic vascular grafts: the biohybrids. Biohybrid or biosynthetic grafts typically consisted of a Dacron prosthesis which had been coated with a film of biological proteins. The biological coating varied in type of protein, means of application and postapplication modification of the proteins. Albumin,[10] gelatin[11] and collagen[12] have been most widely used. These proteins opacify the synthetic surface, lessen platelet deposition and decrease graft porosity (minimizing blood loss at the time of implantation). Because of persistent difficulties with graft thrombosis, especially in the small caliber (< 6 mm diameter) grafts, attempts to modify the graft surface thrombogenicity have been undertaken. Two principal methods have been employed: the adsorption of anticoagulant antithrombolytic molecules to the graft luminal surface and the seeding of the graft with endothelial cells. Anticoagulants or fibrinolytic proteins affixed to the inner surface of grafts have included heparin[13] and urokinase.[14] Endothelial cell seeding techniques are still an actively studied area of research and represent a broad area of graft development. More recently, attempts have been made to affix endothelial growth factors onto the prosthesis in order to promote the growth of the seeded endothelial cells. This represents a combination of the two basic methods of modifying the current biosynthetic grafts: by both adsorbing factors onto the graft surface and seeding the same surface with endothelial cells.[15]

Graft Infection

Since synthetic arterial prostheses are foreign bodies, graft infection, although uncommon, is a serious life and limb threatening problem.[16,17,18] The design of an infection-resistant graft has become an important area of research. Initial experience with passive soaking of the prosthesis prior to implantation was disappointing. The antimicrobial activity of the graft disappeared shortly after restoration of the blood flow. Persistence of the antibiotic activity has been as short as four minutes.[19] Subsequent efforts have focused on binding the antibiotic to the surface of the graft.

Moore and coworkers first reported on the development of such a prosthesis in 1981.[20] They used filamentous velour grafts, to which amikacin was bonded using a collagen retention matrix. These grafts were able to resist infection in a canine model which was challenged with the intravenous injection of a suspension of *Staphylococcus aureus.* Greco and his colleagues[21] reported on a series of experiments in which penicillins and cephalosporins were ionically bonded to Dacron and PTFE grafts. Shue and his associates studied Dacron grafts on which tridodecylmethylammonium chloride (TDMAC) was used to bind oxacillin. Again, these grafts were studied for their ability to resist infections when inoculated with *S. aureus* and were found to be moderately successful.[22] More recent experimentation has focussed on the binding of hydrophobic antibiotics such as rifampin to prosthetic grafts in order to extend the antibiotic coverage.

GRAFT HEALING

Graft healing is thought to occur via two mechanisms interaction with blood elements and interaction with surrounding tissue. Blood elements include proteins, platelets, complement factors and leuko-cytes and monocytes. Serum proteins adsorb onto the graft surface upon contact with the prosthetic wall. The concentration of an adsorbed protein is determined by its blood concentration and its affinity to attach to the graft. Such a phenomenon is dynamic, with proteins of greater affinity eventually displacing those with lower affinity even though these might be present in higher concentrations. This is re-ferred to as the "Vroman effect."[23] Albumin, the most abundant blood protein, is initially the most highly adsorbed protein on the surface of the graft. This is subsequently displaced by fibrinogen, which has a greater affinity. More importantly, fibrinogen is able to bind the GPIIb/IIIa receptor complex on the platelet membrane surface. This in turn may lead to platelet activation.

The activated platelets release various bioactive substances includ-ing chemotactic factors for leukocytes, monocytes, fibroblasts and smooth muscle cells. Platelet derived growth factor (PDGF) is one such substance; it has both chemotactic and mitogenic effects on fibroblasts and smooth muscle cells.[24] Leukocytes and monocytes are further attracted by C5a generated through both classical and alternate path-ways of complement activation, following graft implantation. Leuko-cytes adhere to the fibrin coagulum on the inner surface of the graft and also to the growing endothelial cells across the anastomosis. This is then followed by migration of the neutrophils to the subendothelial tissue where their toxic metabolic products such as superoxide anion (O^{-2}), hydrogen peroxide (H_2O_2) and hydroxyl radicals (HO), in addi-tion to collagenases and proteases, are released. This may delay healing by digesting the forming capsule on the inner surface of the graft. Clowes reported a persistently increased mitotic index in the endothe-lial cell population in the area of pannus ingrowth, perhaps due to ongoing endothelial cell injury. Monocytes are also attracted, activated and differentiate into macrophages which not only act as scavengers but also release substances mediating various aspects of lipoprotein metabolism.

At the graft-tissue interface, healing leads to transanastomotic growth of a pannus of endothelial cells derived from the adjacent vessel. This growth however, is limited to 1-2 cm distance from the anastomosis.[25] Another proposed source of endothelial cells for coating the inner surface of the graft is through transinterstitial capillary ingrowth from the surrounding tissue. This has not been shown to occur in man, but rather in an experimental polytetrafluoroethylene (ePTFE) prosthesis with 60µ internodal distance.[26] It should be noted however, that such transinterstitial growth did not occur in grafts with 30μ internodal distance suggesting that the more porous prostheses are not only well incorporated but also develop better endothelialized surface.

VASCULAR PROSTHESES CURRENTLY IN CLINICAL USE

With the evolution of vascular grafting and the experimental use of various synthetic materials, it became evident that the only materials capable of withstanding stress and able to retain tensile strength were Dacron and Teflon. Dacron became more popular due to its ease of handling, compared to the tightly woven early Teflon graft (which preceded the expanded PTFE).

Various modifications to the fabrication of the Dacron·graft were employed in an attempt to create a prosthesis that would closely mimic the native vessel both in its physical and biological characteristics. Two basic forms of Dacron grafts are manufactured: knitted and woven. The knitted is soft, pliable and easy to handle. It suffers the disadvantage of increased porosity. It is less hemostatic at implantation and requires preclotting, a processing step which is cumbersome and time-consuming. One advantage of the increased porosity is the fact that knitted grafts are better incorporated in the process of healing the newly implanted graft. Another index of graft healing, the development of transinterstitial pseudointima, is more complete when compared to more tightly woven grafts.[27]

Woven grafts, with their low porosity due to the closer spacing of the Dacron fibers are also less pliable. The advantage of the low porosity is an increase in the hemostatic characteristic of the graft: It does not require "preclotting" prior to implantation. This is a distinct advantage in the course of urgent operations such as emergency repair of ruptured aneurysms and in patients with clotting disorders. The drawbacks of these grafts include slightly more difficult handling and slower, less complete incorporation. This has translated into an experimentally demonstrated increase in susceptibility to infection.

A new generation of synthetic grafts appeared attempting to combine the two desired characteristics of pliability and hemostasis, by making a knitted Dacron graft less porous when impregnated with resorbable material such as collagen.[12] The use of biogenic substances in the implanted prosthesis raised the issue of immunogenic reactions and rejection. This however did not appear to be a problem.[28] As a result this became the most widely used Dacron graft for aortic replacement.

Teflon as graft material was reintroduced in a new expanded form of ePTFE and gained popularity due to the improved ease of handling. It became the most widely used graft for distal arterial reconstructions. Its advantages are softness and pliability; moreover, it easily develops an inner capsule coating. The work of Clowes and associates, demonstrated that increasing the porosity of the ePTFE graft from 30μ to 60μ internodal distance in baboons promoted more capillary ingrowth transinterstitially into the inner capsule and more complete endothelialization of the graft.[26]

The search for the "ideal graft" is far from complete and it continues to be an active area of research in both the clinical and experimental fields. The ideal graft: 1) is easy to handle; 2) withstands mechanical strain; 3) does not incite an immune reaction; 4) is nonthrombogenic; 5) resists infection; and 6) is easily manufactured at a reasonable cost.

GRAFT INFECTABILITY: FABRIC AND FABRICATION

The majority of vascular graft infections is thought to occur as the result of direct graft contamination at the time of implantation.[29, 30] This contamination may occur as a break in the course of the sterile technique or as a consequence of placing the graft into a colonized arterial bed. The second postulated mechanism of graft infection involves hematogenous exposure of the graft to bacteria. This so-called bacteremic seeding of a graft is thought to account for delayed graft infections whichare present several years following the actual implantation of a graft.[31] Both the ease of direct inoculation and the success of hematogenous infection of a graft are in part related to the composition and manufacture of the graft. (Table 1)

The materials from which a graft is made and the assembly of these materials into a graft appears to play a significant role in determining the susceptibility of a given graft to infection. Russell et al demonstrated in their canine model that Dacron grafts had a 2.5 times greater incidence of infection, compared to PTFE when implanted in a contaminated field.[32] Schmitt and coworkers also demonstrated that in vivo bacterial adherence was greatest to knitted velour Dacron grafts, followed by woven Dacron and then ePTFE.[33] They attributed this difference to the porous property of the velour knitted grafts and the shielding of the organisms in the interstices of the graft from the host defense mechanisms. They also found that not only the graft material and its structure, but also the organism itself, plays a role in bacterial adherence to the prosthesis. Mucin-producing organisms, such as *Staphylococcus epidermidis*, adhered in greater numbers to the grafts when compared to the nonmucin-producing staphylococci, or the gram negative organisms such as *E. coli.* Mucin is thought to produce a stabilizing matrix bonding the bacteria to the prosthesis. *E. coli* on the other hand has a much more complex cell wall structure with multilayers of lipopolysaccharides and proteins. In addition, it has a special organelle of motility, the flagellum, which might contribute to its ability to attach to a graft.

The pseudointima, which consists of a compacted layer of fibrin that develops as part of graft healing, is thought by some to convey a protective layer against hematogenous graft seeding. In studying the

Table 1. Experimental graft infectability as a function of materials.

AUTHOR (ref)	YEAR	STUDY	RESULTS
Moore (31)	1969	Staph bacteremia and graft infection	Dacron susceptible to IV staph injection
Moore (35)	1971	Effect of antibiotic prophylaxis in preventing bacteremic graft infection	IV antibiotics effective in preventing graft infection rates secondary to bacteremia
Cheek	1974	Antibiotic-soaked grafts in fecally contaminated wounds	Antibiotic-soaked Dacron grafts preferable to aortic autografts in contaminated wounds
Malone & Moore (29)	1975	Effect of pseudointima development on graft infection	Pseudointimal development provides effective protection against bacteremic graft infection
Weber & Lindenauer	1976	Comparison of knitted velour and woven Dacron in susceptibility to percutaneous staph injection	Knitted and velour more resistant after two weeks.
Roon, Malone & Moore (34)	1977	Comparison of knitted Dacron, velour and expanded Teflon in IV staph bacteremia	Earlier, more complete pseudointimal development and better resistance to infection in the velour grafts
Weiss	1977	Comparison of PTFE to Dacron in face of bacteremia	Dacron superior in an infected environment
Moore & Malone (37)	1980	Comparison of Dacron ultralight, velour, IMPRA PTFE, double and gore-tex PTFE in bacteremia	Dacron superior to PTFE in pseudointimal development and resistance to bacteremic infection
Rutledge (36)	1982	Comparison of Rifampin to Cefazolin in PTFE graft infection	Rifampin better antibiotic
Russell et al (32)	1984	Infectability of PTFE vs Dacron grafts in contaminated fields	2.5 times greater incidence of graft infection in Dacron compared to PTFE
Schmitt et al (33)	1986	Bacterial adherence to vascular prostheses	Greatest adherence to Dacron knitted velour, then woven, then ePTFE. Mucin-producing bacteria have greatest adherence

effect of pseudointimal development on bacteremic infectability of vascular prosthetic grafts, Malone and associates studied the rate of infection of knitted Dacron grafts implanted in a canine model, when challenged with an intravenous bolus of *Staphylococcus aureus*.[29] They correlated the resistance to infection with the duration from the time of implantation, and the completeness of the pseudointimal layer. Fifty-four of their 57 ulcerated grafts (95%) were infected, compared to 0 graft infection in the 26 grafts with complete intimal lining. Thus the greater the extent of neointima formation following graft implantation, the greater the resistance to bacteremic seeding. In a subsequent study comparing the degree of neointimal development and bacteremic infection in various grafts, Roon noted the external velour Dacron graft (Sauvage USCI) to be the earliest and most completely covered with a neointima.[34] This was followed by the expanded Teflon graft (IMPRA) and then by the ultra-lightweight knitted Dacron graft (USCI). Furthermore, the rate of graft infection followed the same order, once again correlating the degree of neointimal development to graft infection. The superior result of the velour graft was attributed to the ability of the velour elements to coalesce and capture the fibrin proteins onto the graft surface. Additionally, the velour elements allow improved incorporation of the graft into the fibrous tissue reaction which envelops the graft.

CONCLUSION

Despite major advances in vascular grafting, the search for the ideal graft continues. The ideal material would provide pliability and ease of handling. The design should strike a balance between homeostasis at the time of implantation and adequate porosity to allow transinterstitial ingrowth of protective neointima.

The new generation of biosynthetic grafts combine structural design and attempt to convey biological function to closely mimic the native blood vessel. Even though research in this area is very active, and various grafts resisting thrombosis and infection and capable of enhancing neointimal formation have been developed and experimentally tested, no such graft has been approved for clinical use.

The limitations arise, when extrapolating from the experimental laboratory model to the clinical setting. A positive graft culture need not necessarily signify a clinical graft infection. The relatively high inoculation density of *Staphylococcus aureus* may not be clinically significant. Finally, the healing characteristics of the animal models used are different from those of humans. Canine models develop a thicker, continuous layer of neointima which has not been found to occur in humans. Nevertheless, the encouraging results of various experimental studies of antibiotic-impregnated grafts provide a reason for optimism that such an infection-resistant graft is on the horizon.

REFERENCES

1. Callow A. Historical development of vascular grafts. In: Sawyer PN KM, ed. Vascular grafts. New York: Appleton-Century-Croft, 1978: 5.
2. Gross RE, Hurwitt E, Bill AH et al. Preliminary observations on the use of human arterial grafts in the treatment of certain cardiovascular defects. N Engl J Med 1948; 239: 578.
3. Fisher B, Wild R, Engstrom P et al. Experimental reconstruction of the aortic bifurcation. Surgery 1956; 39: 940.
4. DeBakey ME, Creech O, Cooley DA.. Occlusive disease of the aorta and its treatment by resection and homograft replacement. Ann Surg 1954; 140: 290.
5. Szilagyi DE, Smith R, Overhulse PR. Segmental aortoiliac and femoral arterial occlusion:treatment by resection and arterial graft replacement. JAMA 1955; 157: 426.
6. Warren R. Discussion of paper by Szylagyi DE, Whithcomb JG, Smith RF. Ann Surg 1956; 144: 632.
7. Linton RR. Discussion of paper by DeBakey ME, Crawford ES, Cooley DA, Morris GC: Surgical considerations of occlusive disease of the abdominal aorta and iliac and femoral arteries: Analysis of 803 cases. Ann Surg 1958; 148: 306.
8. Voorhees AB, Jarctski A, Blakemore AH. The use of tubes constructed from Vinyon "N" clot in bridging arterial defects. Ann Surg 1952; 135: 332.
9. Callow AD. Historical overview of experimental and clinical development of vascular Grafts. In: Stanley JC, ed. Biologic and synthetic vascular prostheses. New York: Grune & Stratton, 1982: 11-24.
10. Lyman DJ, Metcalf L, Albo D etal. The effect of chemical structure and surface properties of synthetic polymers on the coagulation of blood.In vivo adsorption of proteins on polymer surfaces. Trans Am Soc Artif Organs 1974; 20: 474-478.
11. Drury JK, Ashton T, Cunningham JD et al. Experimental and clinical experience with a gelatin impregnated Dacron prosthesis. Ann Vasc Surg 1987; 1: 542-547.
12. Quinones-Baldrich WJ, Moore WS, Ziomet S, Chapvil M. Development of a "leak-proof" knitted Dacron vascular prosthesis. J Vasc Surg 1986; 3: 895.
13. Nojiri C, Park K, Grainger DW et al. In vivo nonthrombogenicity of heparin immobilized polymer surfaces. Tran Am Soc Artif Intern Organs 1990; 36: M168-M172.
14. Forster RI, Bernath F. Analysis of urokinase immobilization on the polytetrafluoroethylene vacsular prosthesis. Am J Surg 1988; 156: 130-132.
15. Greisler HP, Klosak J, Dennis JW et al. Biomaterial pretreatment with ECGF to augment endothelial cell proliferation. J Vasc Surg 1987; 2: 393-402.
16. Fry WJ. Vascular prosthesis infections. Surg Clin North Am 1972; 52: 1419-1424.
17. Goldstone J, Moore WS. Infection in vascular prostheses. Am J Surg 1974; 128: 225-233.

18. Jamieson GG, DeWeese J, Rob CG. Infected arterial grafts. Ann Surg 1975; 181: 850-852.

19. Kempczinski RF. Discussion of paper by Moore et al. Arch Surg 1981; 116: 1407.

20. Moore WS, Chvapil M. Sieffert G, Keown K. Development of an infection-resistant vascular prosthesis. Arch Surg 1981; 116: 1403-1407.

21. Greco RS, Harvey RA. The role of antibiotic bonding in the prevention of vascular prosthetic infections. Ann Surg 1982; 195: 168-171.

22. Shue WB, Worosilo SC, Donetz AP et al. Prevention of vascular prosthetic infection with an antibiotic-bonded Dacron graft. J Vasc Surg 1988; 8: 600-605.

23. Vroman L. Methods of investigating protein interaction on artificial and natural surfaces. Annals of The New York Academy of Sciences 1987; 516: 300-305.

24. Greisler HP. Vascular graft healing—interfacial phenomena. In: New Biologic And Synthetic Vascular Prostheses. Austin: R.G. Landes Company, 1-15.

25. Clowes AW, Kirkman T, Clowes MM. Mechanism of arterial graft failure. II. Chronic endothelial and smooth muscle cell proliferation in healing polytetrafluoroethylene prostheses. J Vasc Surg 1986; 3: 877-884.

26. Clowes AW, Kirkman T, Reidy MA. Mechanisms of arterial graft healing. AM J Path 1986; 123: 220-230.

27. Wesolowski SA, Fries C, Karleson CE et al. Porosity: Primary detreminant of the fate of synthetic vacsular grafts. Surgery 1961; 50: 91-96.

28. The Canadian Multicenter Hemashield Study Group. Immunologic response to collagen-impregnated Vascular grafts: A randomized prospective study. J Vasc Surg 1990; 12: 741-746.

29. Malone JM, Moore WS, Campagno G, Bean B. Bacteremic infectability of vascular grafts: The influence of pseudointimal integrity and duration of graft function. Surgrey 1975; 78(2): 211-216.

30. Moore WS, Swanson RJ, Campagna G, Bean B. Pseudointimal development and vascular prosthesis, susceptibility to bacteremic infection. Surg Forum 1974; 25: 250-252.

31. Moore WS, Rosson CT, Hall AD, Thomas AN. Transient bacteremia: A cause of infection in prosthetic vascular grafts. Amer J Surg 1969; 117: 342.

32. Russell WL, Bard R, Krahwinkel DJ, Burns RP. A comparison of graft infectability of Dacron versus PTFE in the canine model. In: Skotnicki SH BFGM Reinaerts H.H.M,, ed. Recent Advances in Vascular Grafting. Gerrards Cross, Buckinghamshire, England: System 4 Associates, 1984: 220-225.

33. Schmitt DD, Bandyk D, Pequet A, Towne J. Bacterial adherence to vascular prostheses. J Vasc Surg 1986; 3: 732-740.

34. Roon AJ, Moore WS, Barton B, Campagna G. Bacteremic infectability: A function of vascular graft material and design. J Surg Res. 1977; 22: 489-498.

35. Moore WS, Rossen CT, Hall AD. Effect of prophylactic antibiotics in preventing bacteremic infection of vacsular prosthesis. Surgery 1971; 69: 825-828.

36. Rutledge RB, Sheretz V, Johnson R. Rifampin and cefazolin as prophylactic agents. Arch Surg 1982; 117: 1164-1165.

37. Moore WS, Malone JM, Keown K. Prosthetic arterial graft material. Infuence on neointimal healing and bacteremic infectibility. Arch Surg 1980; 115: 1379-1383.

38. Rutledge R, Baker V, Shertz R, Johnson G. Rifampin and Cefazolin as prophylactic agents. Arch Surg 1982; 117: 1164-1165.

CHAPTER 5

MODELS OF GRAFT INFECTION DEVELOPMENT AND USE

Hugh A. Gelabert

INTRODUCTION

While the consequences of graft infection are well known, the exact mechanisms which account for these infections remain a mystery. The self-evident notions of contamination and the propagation of bacteria within a host are not necessarily applicable to clinical graft infections. In this simplistic view, graft infections are the result of bacterial contamination, much like the spread of bacteria in a large petri dish. This is not necessarily accurate. The probability of a graft infection resulting from a chance break in sterile technique during the implantation of a vascular prosthesis has not and cannot be clearly assessed.

Evidence that not all bacterial exposure results in graft infection is available from a number of sources. Perhaps the most compelling information is that which is derived from clinical studies which have outlined the incidence of positive bacterial cultures from aneurysmal contents, inguinal nodes and arterial walls.[1,2,3] According to these studies, the range of bacterial contamination of these tissues is between 10 and 30%. At the same time, we know that the incidence of clinical graft infections is much lower. The discrepancy between these two infection rates signifies that either some grafts will be successfully sterilized in the course of treatment with parenteral antibiotics, or that a number of graft infections progress slowly to the clinical stage.

A significant problem in studying graft infections is the relative infrequency of these events. The low incidence of these infections impairs the ability of individuals and institutions to review large numbers of patients. Accordingly, most clinical reviews are either anecdotal experiences or compilations of many disparate experiences. Experimental modeling has allowed investigators to overcome these limitations by permitting the generation and investigation of graft infections as required for study. Experimental modeling has further facilitated the study of graft infection problems by allowing the investigators to control the many variables associated with these problems. Modeling provides a quicker, more reliable method of screening treatments and testing hypothesis related to prosthetic infections. Thus, graft infection models are of vital importance in formulating and testing hypothesis which in turn may yield improved care for these patients.

Despite the many advantages of graft infection modeling, many nuances of the models are not entirely self-evident, and data which they generate must be interpreted strictly in the context of the model and its limitations. When applying information derived from a model to human clinical graft infection problems, it is important to evaluate not only the data but the model itself. If incorrect assumptions lead to the incorrect use of a model, then the wrong conclusions will be reached. The goal of this chapter is to review the use of models in the study of vascular graft infections. The strengths and limitations of the more common models will be outlined along with the rationale for their use. Additionally, the projects which have formed the focus of these experiments will be outlined.

MODELING GRAFT INFECTION

The value of a model is its ability to provide insight into the mechanisms which generate graft infections and to advance the management of graft infections. Specifically, models allow the investigator to control a series of variables associated with graft infections, while focusing on the dependent variables which are under study. This facilitates investigation of graft infections in ways which would be impossible in a human population. It also allows the collection of data in statistically significant numbers. Finally, it permits the application of rigorous methodology so as to exclude the random variables associated with the independent work of any clinicians.

The ideal model is one which is reproducible, simple and readily interpreted. The ideal model should allow an easy comprehension of its relevance to the clinical problem under investigation. The model should yield results which are understandable and may be clearly described in statistical terms. Thus, the data from the best of models are both clinically relevant, statistically significant and have a self-evident quality which imparts certainty in their significance.[4] Finally, the clinical relevance of a graft infection model is important since the ambition of these models is the resolution of a clinical problem. Models which are not clearly defined with regards to the clinical problem may risk insignificance by virtue of failing to address the question which they originally sought to answer.

The statistical impact of a model resides in its ability to be analyzed with simple and clear statistical methods. The primary factor which will limit the statistical significance of any model is the design of the experiment. Experimental design should be as simple as necessary to provide answers to the questions being sought. The design should allow the collection of data in such a manner that will be simple to quantify and to analyze. Semi-quantitative results are difficult to interpret and subject to considerable error.

THE PRIMARY MODELS

Experimental investigation of prosthetic graft infections has resulted in the development of several models which have become standards in the study of graft infection. These models have been employed in the course of development of graft materials, the testing of antibiotics and the application of antibiotics to grafts. The topics which have been addressed by means of these models include the pathophysiology of graft infections, the interaction between the host and the implanted graft, techniques of managing graft infections and the development of antibiotic bonded prosthetic vascular grafts.

The three types of models which may be reasonably named as the standards in the investigation of graft infections include: the in vitro testing of grafts and organisms, the subcutaneous implantation techniques; and the large animals graft implantation experiments. Each of these models has been extensively used in a variety of manners so as to mimic certain aspects of graft infections. The models differ significantly in their ability to reproduce a clinical graft infection, yet each has certain advantages which make it valuable.

IN VITRO MODELS

The in vitro approach to questions pertaining graft infection has found principal application with regards to testing of the prosthetic grafts: specifically the bonding of antibiotics of these grafts and the

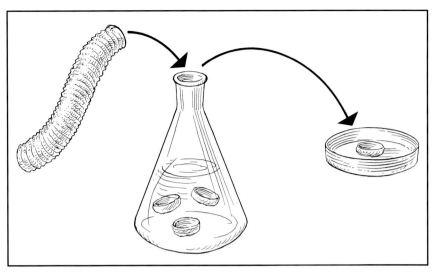

Fig. 1. Illustration of an in vitro model commonly used in the study of antibiotic binding. A bonded graft is placed in elution flask. Following the period of elution, a segment of graft is placed on an agar plate for sensitivity disk testing in order to determine the residual antibiotic activity.

subsequent antibacterial properties of these bound grafts.[5,6,7,8,9,10,11,12] The in vitro models allow the rapid screening of materials and pharmaceuticals in a rigidly controlled environment. In vitro testing allows quantification of many variables which might not otherwise be assayed in in vivo trials. (Fig. 1)

The typical in vitro models consist of pairings of several standard assays in order to reach a desired endpoint. The principal assays employed are bacterial cultures, disk sensitivity assays and in-flask elution or soaking of grafts. Additional assays occasionally employed include nucleotide measurement of antibiotic concentrations, microscopic evaluations of graft surfaces and phage typing of bacteria.

Most of the in vitro models begin with the preparation of a vascular prosthesis by binding an antibiotic to it, then subjecting it to test conditions. The efficacy of the binding itself may be tested. In the elution experiments, the bonded graft is immersed in a solution which is designed to mimic human serum.[6,10,12] The solutions are frequently saline based and may contain serum proteins. The graft is maintained in the elution solutions for a number of days. Periodically, a segment of graft is tested for retention of the antibiotic. This may be accomplished by plating the section of graft on an agar plate onto which bacteria have been inoculated. This results in a "disk sensitivity" type assay. The bioavailable antibiotic on the graft disk will inhibit the growth of bacteria in a perimeter surrounding the grafts. The area of growth inhibition is directly proportional to the concentration of antibiotic in the graft.

A variation on the elution technique uses the elutant solution for the microbiological assays. In this scheme, the infected-bonded graft is washed. The wash solution is collected and plated onto an agar plate or inoculated in to a tube of sterile broth. Then a count is made of the number of replicating organisms.

Another standard means of evaluating a graft in vitro is an assay of the ability of the graft to inhibit the adherence of viable bacteria onto the graft surface.[7,8,9, 11] In such a study, the graft is first bonded with its antibiotic. The bonded graft is then immersed in a bacterial solution for a given period of time. Next, the graft is washed to rinse off any loosely adherent organisms. Finally segments of the grafts are plated onto an agar plate or immersed into sterile nutrient broth. The final step involves assaying the number of bacteria found on the plate or in the broth. This is compared with the same result following the use of a nonbonded graft.

The bioavailability of antibiotics which have be bonded to grafts is an important subject of study since the efficacy of the bonded graft is directly related to the amount of bioavailable antibiotic. It is the bioavailable antibiotic which would be expected to produce a clinical reduction of the graft infection. Bioavailability studies have labeled the antibiotic bonded to a graft and compared this to the amount which is expressed in a disk sensitivity assay. One study demonstrated that about 20% of the total bonded antibiotic is biologically active.[5]

If the advantage of the in vitro modeling is that rapid, exact experiments may be performed with the precision and control of a laboratory, the principal drawback is that these experiments do not closely mimic the human clinical experience. The in vitro testing of grafts and bacteria cannot replicate the balance between the inoculum and the host defenses. It is the complex interaction between the graft, the invading bacteria and the host antibacterial agents which determines the outcome of a graft infection.

SUBCUTANEOUS AND INTRAMUSCULAR POUCH MODELS

The use of subcutaneous and intramuscular pouches in the investigation and development of antibiotic bonded vascular grafts has been and continues to be a popular model.[5,6,10,13,14] In essence, this model involves the creation of a small pocket either under the skin or between the muscle bundles of the host animal. Typically these experiments are performed on small mammals such as rats of guinea pigs. A small disk of antibiotic-bonded graft material is placed into the pouch for later retrieval. The experiments have the advantages of involving host defense mechanisms and thus begin to simulate the biological interactions which are the essence of graft infection problems. (Fig. 2)

The most common use for the pouch experiments is the testing of antibiotic binding techniques. The tests include both elution type experiments and infection resistance experiments. In the elution experiments, the disk of bonded graft is tested periodically using disk sensitivity type methods. Thus, experimenter hope to discover when the antibiotic was biologically eluted from the graft. The second general type of pouch experiment involves infecting the bonded graft at the time of its implantation. The disk is then removed after a given period of time and cultured in an attempt to identify any bacteria which may have survived.

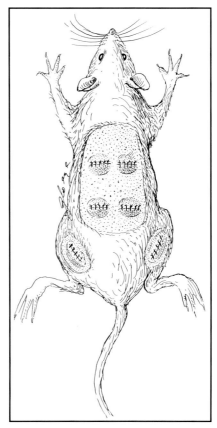

Fig. 2. Illustration of a pouch type model. In this experiment, a disk of graft material is treated with antibiotic and placed into a subcutaneous or intramuscular pouch. This may be simultaneously infected. The pouch is closed and the graft retrieved following a period of inoculation. The recovered graft is then tested for the presence of bacteria, or the retention of antibiotic.

The principal advantages of this system is its low cost and the consequent ability to perform a significantly large number of trials in the course of an experimental protocol.

It also has the advantage of involving the biological mechanism which are at play in the clinical situation which the experiment addresses. The subcutaneous disk method has been very convenient in studies which have tried to determine which antibiotic, or which antibiotic binding method, is most effective in treatment of a graft infection. These experiments allow screening of fairly large numbers of grafts, organisms and antibiotic binding techniques. They are relatively inexpensive and yield results in short order, making this an attractive experimental model.

The main disadvantage of this system is that the environment in which the grafts are tested is not at all similar to the exposure to which the grafts are subjected in clinical use. While this model has been used in an attempt to study the elution of antibiotics from vascular grafts, the validity of these results is in question. The cellular kinetics and fluid dynamics of an intramuscular pouch are not at all similar to what is found within the vascular system. Grafts in this model are not exposed to flowing blood, plasma proteins and cellular elements of both the blood or the arterial wall. Accordingly, experiments which are intended to test vascular grafts with regards to the retention of antibiotic, or the ability to resist infection, may not be valid.

Another objection frequently voiced regarding the pouch models is the use of multiple trials in one subject. Typically, several pouches are fashioned in the subject animal. These are then used simultaneously in the experiment. The principal concern in this situation is that the course of one trial may alter the results of another trial. In essence: It is unreasonable in this situation to assume that the trials are truly independent. Thus the outcomes may not reflect the expectation that each trial is a separate and independent event.

While this concern is more of a theoretical than a conclusively demonstrated one, it persists. Experiments which test the resistance of a grafts implanted against a bacterial challenge are of particular concern since the result of any particular trial may in fact reflect cross-contamination rather than an actual graft failure.

CANINE MODELS

Most experimental studies of graft infection have relied upon canine vascular graft models. The essence of these experiments is the implantation of a vascular prosthesis into a dog and the subsequent bacterial challenge of the prosthesis.[15,16,17,18,19,20,21] The ultimate goals are to study the pathogenesis of graft infections, the efficacy of antibiotic bonded grafts in resisting infection and the management of graft infections. (Fig. 3)

These goals are most often addressed in the context of one of two types of experiments. First is the direct bacterial infection of a prosthesis by the application of a known organism directly onto the graft or infusion into the host bloodstream. These experiments may be referred to as primary graft challenge experiments since the primary or first implanted graft is challenged by the inoculation of bacteria. The second type of experiment is the implantation of the graft into the bed of a prior graft infection. These experiments have been referred to as "in-line replacement" of infected grafts.

Primary graft challenge experiments have been widely used in the development of bonding techniques for the application of antibiotics to grafts. The prototypical format of these experiments involves the application of the antibiotic to the graft, the subsequent implantation of the graft and finally the contamination of the graft. The grafts are allowed to incubate for a period of time and are recovered and tested for the presence of organisms or antibiotic activity. Of particular importance in these experiments is the fact that the graft which is implanted is sterile until it is contaminated, and that the method of contamination is controlled (either direct application of bacteria or the infusion of bacteria). The subsequent infection should be the result of the bacterial challenge. If the infected graft is the primary graft, then the subsequent infection is a primary graft infection. This experimental format allows one to infect with a known pathogen, at a known point in time, and to recover the graft at a specific point following the infectious challenge. Consequently, these are the principal variables which are studied in these experiments.

In-line replacement experiments are designed to provide a more severe challenge to the antibiotic-laden graft.[22,23,24,25] In these experiments, the subjects undergo arterial reconstruction (usually the abdominal aorta) with a standard vascular graft which is contaminated at the time of implantation. Following a period of incubation, the infection is confirmed, the first graft is removed, the infected tissues are debrided and the antibiotic bonded graft is implanted into the bed of the infected graft. The second graft is then recovered following a period of implantation;

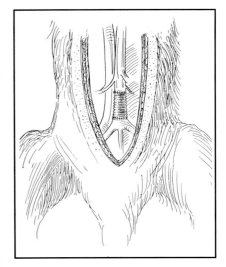

Fig. 3. Illustration of a canine graft model. In this experiment, the graft is implanted in the infrarenal aorta. It may be inoculated with bacteria by direct application or hematogenoulsy. The graft is allowed to incubate, then retrieved and tested for the presence of bacterial organisms.

it then may be tested for the presence of infectious agents and its antibacterial properties.

These studies are directed towards the development of effective methods of treating graft infections by replacing an infected graft with an antibiotic bonded graft. The experiments which have been performed to date suggest that this option may come to fruition with improvements in the use of bonded and adjunctive antibiotics. The best results with these in-line replacements have suggested that the secondary infection rates may be in the range of 10-20%.[35] This is comparable to current management with remote bypass grafting for prosthetic infections.

VARIABLES

It is important to recognize that graft infection models will typically incorporate several specific variables. The most commonly studied variables include the grafts used, the antibiotic which is used to protect the grafts and the method by which these antibiotics are applied to the graft. Additional considerations in these experiments include the infectious organisms, the timing and route of bacterial challenge and the timing of the infection. Other variations in the models have included the location into which the grafts are placed and the methods of evaluating the outcome of the challenge.

GRAFTS: USE OF ANTIBIOTICS AND ANTIBIOTIC BINDING

The ability of a given graft to resist infection has been the subject of experimental investigation. Some authors have suggested that certain grafts offer superior resistance to infection. This has been demonstrated in experiments where grafts are exposed to bacterial challenges and subsequently treated with antibiotics. Some authors have been able to document a reduced incidence of graft infection by double velour grafts.[18] Other reports have concluded that PTFE may be more resistant to infection than the Dacron grafts.[26]

The resolution of this paradox may rest in the timing of infectious challenges and the degree of incorporation and endothelial covering of the grafts at the time of challenge.[15,18] Different grafts may be superior in withstanding infection via different routes. A well healed and well incorporated Dacron double velour graft will withstand a hematogenous bacterial challenge better than a PTFE graft. On the other hand, bacteria directly applied onto a freshly implanted graft are less able to adhere to PTFE than to Dacron grafts. This has been cited in support of using PTFE grafts in trauma surgery, where some degree of wound contamination would be suspected as the prime source of graft infection.

Modeling has been used to study the efficacy of antibiotics in preventing and treating graft infections. The question of which antibiotic to use and how to employ it has been the essence of most graft infection work during the past three decades. The antibiotics selected may be studied with regards to its properties: solubility, antibacterial spectrum of activity and the incidence of bacterial resistance on exposure. The methods of binding the antibiotics to a graft and the reasons to use one antibiotic over another are the subjects of other sections of this monograph and will not be covered further here.

ORGANISMS

Since most clinical graft infections are produced by gram positive organisms, the majority of graft infection models have used the same organisms for experimental purposes. The most common bacteria studied have been gram-positive organisms such as *Staphylococcus aureus* and *Staphylococcus epidermidis*. Some investigators have worked with gram-negative organisms such as *Klebsiella pneumonia* [20] or *Escherichia coli* [26] and others have used combinations of these gram-positive and gram-negative bacteria.[27] The choice of organism is significant since it affects the virulence of the resultant infection. It will also affect the outcome of the experiment since some organisms are more difficult to culture and others are more difficult to eradicate. It is conceivable that an experiment using an organism such as *S. epidermidis* may underestimate the incidence of infection since these organisms are frequently not readily grown from graft samples or wound swabs. Towne and his associates have devoted considerable effort to improving the detection of these bacteria. They have discovered techniques which significantly improve the detection of graft infections caused by *S. epidermidis*.[23,28,29] Still the difficulty in culturing these bascteria limits their use in graft-infection models.

A second example of the importance of organisms in the outcome of an experiment is the synergistic effect of certain organisms in producing a necrotizing infection. Ney and associates used both *E. coli* and *S. aureus* to produce graft infections following arterial reconstructions in dogs.[19] They noted necrotizing arterial infections and anastomotic disruptions as a consequence of the synergistic effect of the gram-positive and gram-negative organisms. Should arterial anastomotic disruption be one of the clinical indications used in evaluating the presence or absence of a graft infection, then the organisms employed will have a significant impact on the expected frequency this event. Thus it is an important consideration in the planning of an experiment.

METHOD OF INOCULATION

The methods of inoculating a graft provide a significant differentiation between graft experiments. The route of inoculation is important since one of the prerequisites of a successful model is its ability to mimic the clinical problem in question. In actual practice, the principal means used to inoculate grafts are either direct application of a bacterial suspension to the graft, or the intravenous infusion of a bacterial suspension into the host organism. These two methods of contaminating a graft reflect the principal theories of graft infection: direct intraoperative contamination with bacteria or hematogenous infection from any one of a number of sources. Finally, a few experiments have challenged grafts by implanting these into the bed of a prior graft infection.

The method of inoculation may significantly affect the experimental outcome since suboptimal bacterial challenges may fail to infect grafts. The question of whether there exists a supramaximal inoculum has not been addressed. How many organisms are required to infect a prosthesis has not been extensively studied. In experiments where grafts were infected by directly applying bacteria to the graft surface after implantation, Weber and colleagues found that higher inoculum (1×10^5 versus 1×10^6) resulted in a greater rate of infection.[30]

The number of organisms required to infect a graft appears to vary with the route of inoculation. Some evidence would suggest that the number of organisms required to produce a graft infection via hematogenous seeding of a graft may be greater than that required for direct contamination. This is reflected in the experiments which use 1×10^8 organisms for hematogenous challenges.[31,32,33,21] Most experiments which produce graft infections by means of direct contamination of the grafts use bacterial concentrations from 1×10^{3}[34] to 1×10^{8}.[19,27,29] Recent experimental data suggests that the minimal inoculum required to produce a graft infection when applied directly to a vascular prosthesis is considerably lower. Colburn and associates have presented data indicating that arterial prosthetic grafts were reliably infected with an inoculum of 1×10^2 *S. aureus*.[35] Thus an inoculum which is sufficient to cause a graft infection by one route, may not be insufficient via the other. The lower limits of bacterial contamination necessary for the generation of a graft infection are not well defined.

TIMING OF INFECTION

Temporal variables are of critical importance since these relate directly to the incorporation of the graft, the ingrowth of neointima and to the infectability of the graft. Moore and associates discovered that a graft implanted for four weeks is better able to resist infection than one implanted for a shorter period of time.[15] They attributed this to the in growth of endothelial cells forming a neointima within the graft. They were able to demonstrate that the infections correlated with the development of a neointima and that this was a time-dependent event. Further, infections occurred in "older" grafts when there was an im,pediment of the endothelial ingrowth.

In another project, these investigators studied the infectability of grafts as a function of their incorporation.[18] The incorporation of Dacron grafts and PTFE grafts were compared. The double velour graft was found to be superior with regards to its incorporation and also demonstrated the lowest incidence of infection after a two-month period of implantation. The improved protection against infection was thought to reflect the superior incorporation of the graft.

In an similar experiment, Weber and colleagues investigated the local infection of vascular prostheses.[30] In this experiment, they inoculated grafts after three distinct periods following implantation. The inoculation was done by direct injection of the organisms onto the graft surface. They discovered that the type graft, the size of the inoculum and the period of implantation all were significant variables in determining the incidence of infection. Double velour grafts withstood the challenge better than standard woven or knitted grafts. Further, they determined the lower the inoculum and the longer the implantation period prior to inoculum, the lower the infection rate.

ADJUNCTIVE USE OF ANTIBIOTICS

The choice of which antibiotics and how long they should be used in preventing graft infections have been the focus of several investigations. The general approach has been to implant a graft, then subject the host to a bacterial challenge. This is followed by treatment with antibiotics after which the graft is recovered and studied for evidence of infection. Using this method, Rutledge and colleagues found rifampin to be superior to cephazolin in reducing the number of graft infections.[34] Other groups such as those of Greco[36] and Moore[37] have distinguished themselves in the search for antibiotics to use both in bonding with grafts and as adjuncts to the management of graft infection.

GRAFT LOCATION

The choice of which arteries to reconstruct with the prosthetic graft is significant since it may affect the results of the experiment. While the standard arterial reconstruction is the replacement of the infrarenal aorta in the dog, several investigators have used other vessels. Reconstructions of the dog iliac, carotid and femoral arteries have been reported. When investigators use the patency of a graft as presumptive evidence of graft infection, then the location of the graft is of critical importance. The expected patency of grafts at various locations is not equal and spontaneous thrombosis is more likely in the more peripheral positions (femoral, carotid).

The location in which the graft is implanted will also be significant in determining which type of experiment may be performed. An in-line replacement may be accomplished in the abdominal aortic position, but would probably not be feasible in a femoral or carotid position. The location of the graft may be significant with regards to the contamination of the graft. Much like the clinical picture of graft infection, grafts placed into the inguinal region of the dogs may be subject to more probable spontaneous infection than those placed within the abdominal cavity. While this has not been established conclusively, some investigators consider the possibility sufficiently significant that they would not want to risk this problem. Accordingly, one should avoid these reconstructions in experimental designs.

CONCLUSIONS

Prosthetic vascular graft infections remain a relatively uncommon, but singularly difficult problem. The associated morbidity and mortality make these cases both undesirable and fraught with risk. Under such circumstances it is reasonable that both physicians and patients are unwilling to undergo experimental or investigational procedures without the benefit of preliminary laboratory investigations. Modeling of graft infections provides the vehicle by which we can investigate and generate innovative approaches to the problems of graft infection in preparation for clinical application.

The future directions of research in the management and prophylaxis of graft infections clearly will involve more fundamental studies of the interaction of organisms, host and graft. The application of more in vitro experimentation is to be expected. Further, the use of the powerful techniques of molecular biology in a attempt to understand the complex signaling between the host leukocytes in the presence of infectious agents is to be anticipated. Also, the mechanisms by which a prosthesis may inhibit the complete resolution of an infection may lend itself to similar study. Finally, the question of why some grafts become infected while others do not is unanswered and invites studies into the resistance of hosts towards the infection.

The use of molecular biology and cell culture techniques in the generation of new hybrid grafts where cellular elements are seeded onto the prosthetic materials are beginning to emerge as the new frontier of graft infection research. Improved resistance to hematogenous infection has been demonstrated at intervals of up to 10-12 months.

While many areas of surgical endeavor have been successfully investigated in vitro using the techniques of bacterial culture, cell culture, molecular biology and recombinant genetics, the same cannot be said of vascular prosthetic graft infections. Animal models have been essential to the study of graft infection for a number of reasons. The complex interaction of host, prosthesis and pathogens remains largely a mystery. The elements which are involved are only partly known. Animal models allow the examination of these elements in an environment which most closely resembles the actual clinical problem.

REFERENCES

1. Schwartz J, Powell T, Burnham S, Johnson G Jr. Culture of abdominal aortic aneurysm contents: An additional series. Arch Surg 1987; 122: 777-780.
2. Malone J, Lalka S, McIntyre K, Bernhard V, Pabst T. The necessity for long term antibiotic therapy with positive arterial wall cultures. J Vasc Surg 1988; 8: 262-268.
3. Wakefiled T, Pierson C, Schaberg D et al. Artery, periarterial adipose tissue and blood microbiology during vascular reconstructive surgery: Perioperative and early postoperative observations. J Vasc Surg 1990; 11: 624-628.
4. Rutledge R, Burnham SJ, Johnson G Jr. The use of animal models in studying vascular graft infection. Contemp Surg 1984; 24(June): 61-65.
5. Henry R, Harvey R, Greco R. Antibiotic bonding to vascular prosthesis. J Thor Cardiovasc Surg 1981; 82: 272-277.
6. Harvey R, Alcid D, Greco R. Antibiotic bonding to polytetrafluoroethylene with tridodecylammonium chloride. Surgery 1982; 92: 504-512.
7. Rosenman J, Pearce W, Kempczinski R. Bacterial adherence to vascular grafts after in vitro bacteremia. J Surg Res 1985; 38: 648-655.
8. Webb L, Myers R, Cordell A et al. Inhibition of bacterial adhesion by antibacterial surface pretreatment of vascular prosthesis. J Vasc Surg 1986; 4: 16-21.
9. Schmitt D, Bandyk D, Pequet A, Towne J. Bacterial adherence to vascular prostheses. J Vasc Surg 1986; 3: 732-740.
10. Modak S, Sampath L, Fox C et al. A new method for the direct incorporation of antibiotic in prosthetic vascular grafts. Surg Gynecol Obstet 1987; 164: 143-147.
11. Siverhus D, Schmitt D, Edmiston C et al. Adherence of mucin and non-mucin producing staphylococci to preclotted and albumin-coated velour knotted vascular

grafts. Surgery 1990; 107: 613-619.

12. Chervu A, Moore W, Chvapil M, Henderson T. Efficacy and duration of antistaphylococcal activity comparing three antibiotics bonded to Dacron vascular grafts with a collagen release system. J Vasc Surg 1991; 13: 897-901.

13. Richardson R, Pate J, Wolf R et al. The outcome of antibiotic-soaked arterial grafts in guinea pig wounds contaminated with *E coli* or *S aureus*. J Thor Cardiovasc Surg 1970; 59: 635-637.

14. Prahlad A, Harvey R, Greco R. Diffusion of antibiotics from a polytetraethylene-benzalkonium surface. Am Surg 1981; 47: 515-518.

15. Malone J, Moore W, Campagna G, Bean B. Bacteremic infectability of vascular grafts: The influence of pseudointimal integrity and duration of graft function. Surgery 1975; 78: 211-216.

16. Weiss J, Lorenzo F, Campbell C. The behavior if infected arterial prosthesis of expanded polytetrafluoroethylene (Gore-Tex). J Thor Cardiovasc Surg 1977; 73(4): 630-636.

17. Greco R, Harvey R, Henry R, Prahlad A. Prevention of graft infection by antibiotic bonding. Surg Forum 1980; 31: 29-30.

18. Moore W, Malone J, Keown K. Prosthetic arterial graft material. Arch Surg 1980; 115: 1379-1383.

19. Ney A, Kelly P, Tsukayama D, Burrick M. Fibrin glue-antibiotic suspension in the prevention of prosthetic graft infection. J Trauma 1990; 30: 1000-1006.

20. Kinney E, Bandyk D, Seabrook G et al. Antibiotic-Bonded PTFE Vascular Grafts: The effect of silver antibiotic on bioactivity following implantation. J Surg Res 1991; 50: 430-435.

21. Chervu A, Moore W, Gelabert H et al. Prevention of graft infection by use of prosthesis bonded with a rifampin/collagen release system. J Vasc Surg 1991; 14(4): 521-525.

22. Greco R, Trooskin S, Donetz A, Harvey R. The application of antibiotic bonding to the treatment of established vascular prosthetic infection. Arch Surg 1985; 120: 71-75.

23. Bergamini T, Bandyk D, Govostis D et al. Infection in vascular prosthesis caused by bacterial biofilms. J Vasc Surg 1988; 7: 21-30.

24. Martin L, Harris J, Fehr D et al. Vascular prosthetic infection with Staphylococcus epidermidis: Experimental study of pathogenesis and therapy. J Vasc Surg 1989; 9: 464-471.

25. Vetsch R, Bandyk D, Schmitt D et al. Anastomotic tensile strength following in-situ replacement of an infected abdominal aortic graft. Arch Surg 1989; 124: 425-428.

26. Shah P, Ito K, Clauss R et al. Expanded microporous polytetrafluoroethylene (PTFE) grafts in contaminated wounds: experimental and clinical study. J Trauma 1983; 23: 1030-1033.

27. Shenk J, Ney A, Tsykayama D, Olson ME, Bubrick M. Tobramycin-adhesive in preventing and treating PTFE vascular graft infections. J Surg Res 1989; 47: 487-492.

28. Tollefson D, Bandyk D, Kaebnick H et al. Surface biofilm disruption. Arch Surg 1987; 122: 38-43.

29. Bergamini T, Bandyk D, Govostis D et al. Identification of *Staphylococcus epidermidis* vascular graft infections: A comparison of culture techniques. J Vasc Surg 1989; 9: 665-670.

30. Weber T, Lindenauer S, Miller T et al. Focal infection of aortofemoral prostheses. Surgery 1976; 79: 310-312.
31. Wakefiled T, Schaberg D, Pierson C et al. Treatment of established prosthetic vascular graft infection with antibiotics preferentially concentrated in leucocytes. Surgery 1987; 102: 8-14.
32. Leport C, Goen-Brissonniere O, Lebrault C et al. Experimental colonization of a polyester vascular graft with *Staphylococcus aureus*. A quantitative and morphological study. J Vasc Surg 1988; 8: 1-9.
33. Keller J, Falk J, HS B, Silberstein E, Kempczinski R. Bacterial infectability of chronically implanted endothelial cell-seeded expanded polytetrafluoroethylene vascular grafts. J Vasc Surg 1988; 7: 524-530.
34. Rutledge R, Baker V, Shertz R, Johnson G. Rifampin and cefazolin as prophylactic agents. Arch Surg 1982; 117: 1164-1165.
35. Colburn MD, Moore WS, Gelabert HA et al. Use of an antibiotic-bonded graft for in-situ reconstruction following prosthetic graft infections. J Vasc Surg 1992; (submitted).
36. Greco R, Harvey R, Smilow P, Tesoriero J. Prevention of vascular prosthetic infection by a benzalkonium-oxacillin bonded polytetrafluoroethylene graft. Surg Gynecol Obstet 1982; 155: 28-32.
37. Moore W, Chvapil M, Seiffert G, Keown K. Development of an infection-resistant vascular prosthesis. Arch Surg 1981; 116: 1403-1407.

CHAPTER 6

DEVELOPMENT AND RESULTS OF ANTIBIOTIC-IMPREGNATED VASCULAR GRAFTS

Hugh A. Gelabert
Michael D. Colburn

INTRODUCTION

The rationale behind the development of an antibiotic bonded graft is that it may reduce the incidence of graft infections and perhaps allow improved management of established graft infections. The notion of binding antibiotics to a graft is dependent on two ideas: First that a prolonged antibiotic presence in the vicinity of the newly placed graft will effectively combat incipient graft infections; second, that the graft is most vulnerable to infection during the weeks following its implantation. The goal of bonding antibiotics to grafts is to provide a prolonged, gradual release of antibiotic in the vicinity of the graft. This should effectively reduce the incidence of new graft infections. In management of established graft infections, it may allow more direct surgical approaches and improved clinical outcomes.

The purpose of a bonding agent is two-fold. First, the agent serves to seal the graft, reducing its porosity. The textile in synthetic Dacron in particular, contains large interstices which leak after implantation into the vascular system. Prior application of a bonding agent to the prosthetic surface essentially eliminates this "leaking" and greatly facilitates implantation of the graft. Second, the bonding agent serves as a method of temporarily attaching an antibiotic to the graft surface.

The two main routes by which prosthetic vascular grafts are be-lieved to become infected are direct contamination and bacteremic seeding. Therefore, it follows that the clinical success of an antibiotic protected prosthesis will largely be determined by its ability to resist infection by these mechanisms. Direct contamination most commonly occurs during the operation, either from intestinal translocation or breaks in sterile surgical technique. Theoretically, bacteremic contami-nation could occur at any time following implantation. However, in experimental models it has been difficult to document infectability of a healed vascular prosthesis.[1] It appears that, like direct contamination, infection of a prosthetic graft by bacteremic seeding is also more likely to occur in the early perioperative period. Thus, although clinically there is a long latent period before the onset of graft sepsis,[2,3] it is likely that the origin of most cases of graft infection is related to contamina-tion which occurs at the time of graft implantation. The prosthesis is colonized early, before an intimal lining is formed, but the infection remains indolent. Later, clinical graft sepsis occurs when the immune balance has been compromised.

It has been postulated that protecting a prosthesis in the perioperative period and allowing adequate healing to occur, may reduce the inci-dence of subsequent graft infection. Because the experimental data suggests that complete healing of a vascular prosthesis takes several weeks, it is critical that any antibiotic protected graft retain its antimi-crobial activity for at least a similar duration. The antibiotic/bonding agent combination must therefore be capable of releasing the antimi-crobial agent slowly. The important components of any system include the graft itself, the bonding method and the antibiotic agent incorpo-rated into the prosthesis. Each component will contribute to the overall elution properties of the completed graft. A complete discussion related to the merits of the various types of graft material, as well as the appropriate choice of an antibiotic agent, appear elsewhere in this monograph. This chapter will therefore specifically address the benefits and drawbacks of the available types of bonding agents. Finally, we review the literature regarding the reported experience using each method.

BONDING OF ANTIBIOTICS TO A PROSTHETIC VASCULAR GRAFT

Experimentally, several substances have been used as bonding agents for the purpose of attaching antibiotics to vascular prostheses. These include: heavy metals such as silver nitrate,[4-6] the surfactants tridodecylmethylammonium chloride (TDMAC) and benzalkonium chloride,[5-12] chemical glues such as *N*-butyl-2-cyanoacrylate,[13] as well as biological proteins.[14-17] One convenient way to categorize these techniques for discussion is by separating them according to the method by which the antibiotic is attached to the graft material. These methods include passive absorption, topical application, ionic bonding, as well as simple retention by the bonding agent.

PASSIVE ABSORPTION

Passive absorption is a technique by which antibiotics are applied to a vascular graft simply by soaking the prosthesis in a solution containing the antimicrobial agent. This soaking medium can be composed of either a crystalloid solution, or a colloid such as whole blood. Soaking a graft in a crystalloid antimicrobial solution relies solely on the absorption of the antibiotic agent onto the textile material of the prosthesis. Preclotting a graft with blood which has been mixed with an antibiotic has the advantage of combining passive absorption by the textile, with partial retention bonding by the fibrin coating.

TOPICAL APPLICATION

Topical antimicrobial application is a simple method of graft protection which involves the local incorporation of an antibiotic within an agent which is topically applied to the graft. The implanted graft is 'sealed' by coating the external surface and the anastomoses, with a chemical or endogenous protein glue. Chemical glues have the disadvantage of imparting some degree of tissue toxicity. On the other hand, they tend to be more stable than biodegradable proteins. This may contribute to a longer duration of protection from bacterial contamination. One theoretical problem with the topical application of an antibiotic coating is the failure to protect the luminal surface of the graft. One might expect that, while this method may be effective in preventing infection due to direct contamination, bacteremic challenges would be relatively unaffected. Validation of these potential concerns awaits the completion of conclusive experimental studies.

DIRECT IONIC BONDING

Direct bonding of an antibiotic with a heavy metal such as silver nitrate has been shown to produce a stable impregnated graft.[5] Surfactant bonding agents, such as TDMAC and benzalkonium chloride, are also effective and have been studied extensively.[5-12,18] These compounds are positively charged substances which can easily be absorbed onto a prosthetic surface. The coated graft then serves as a cationic anchor for the binding of any negatively charged antibiotic. A theoretical concern regarding this system is the potential thrombogenic effect of the implanted graft. Once the ionically bound antibiotic eludes away from the graft, the positively charged coating remains and may serve to activate circulating clotting mechanisms. Also, concerns have been raised regarding the potential in vivo toxicity of some of the heavy metal bonding agents.

RETENTION

Passive absorption, topical application and ionic bonding of an antibiotic to the prosthetic surface all suffer due to the weakness of the chemical bond. This property ultimately limits the duration of antimicrobial activity which can be achieved using these methods. Covalent bonding of the antibiotic agent, on the other hand, often requires alteration of the molecular configuration of the agent which may interfere with its biological activity. These problems have led to the concept of binding of the antibiotic agent by simple molecular retention. In this method, the antimicrobial drug is trapped by a molecular size disparity between the bonding agent and the antibiotic compound. To avoid the potential toxicity of heavy metals and chemical glues, attention has been focused on the use of biological proteins for the purpose of antibiotic retention.

In our laboratory, we have tested the efficacy of combining several antibiotics with a Dacron graft based on a collagen release system. In this system, the antibiotic is first mixed with a collagen solution and then layered onto an otherwise untreated prosthesis. After minimally cross-linking the collagen/antibiotic coating with formalin vapor, the antibiotic becomes trapped within the interstices of the collagen protein fibers and is nearly completely retained even following aqueous soaking. Because collagen is a biodegradable protein, after implantation of the treated graft into the host circulation, the collagen is gradually degraded by host enzymatic systems which slowly releases the antibiotic into the surrounding tissues. The rate of release of the antibiotic is proportional to the concentration of the antibiotic in the graft and the rate of enzymatic digestion of the collagen impregnated into the graft. Experimentally, this process has produced high tissue levels of antibiotic activity for a prolonged interval.

LITERATURE REVIEW: EXPERIMENTAL RESULTS USING ANTIBIOTIC-IMPREGNATED GRAFTS

Research into the development of an infection resistant vascular graft has been conducted by several investigators. These efforts have ranged from passive coating of grafts with antimicrobial agents, to covalently bonding the antibiotics using a variety of bonding materials. (Table 1) Unfortunately, differences in antibiotic doses, tested organisms and methods of evaluation make comparison of these bonding techniques difficult. The purpose of this section is to review the literature with regards to the experimental data supporting the use of each of these methods. Again, it is convenient to analyze this work according to the technique of antimicrobial bonding employed.

PASSIVE ABSORPTION

The first reports of protecting a prosthetic graft by passive soaking with a antibiotic solution appeared in the 1970s. One of the earliest of these reports was authored by Richardson and associates.[19] In this study, control and antibiotic protected 0.5 cm by 0.5 cm pieces of Dacron grafts were implanted into previously infected subcutaneous wounds on the backs of guinea pigs. The antibiotic treated experimental grafts were presoaked for 15 minutes in a 10% solution. After eight days, the grafts were removed and evaluated for their ability to grow bacteria on appropriate culture media. The results demonstrated that only 15% (6 of 40) of the treated grafts were infected compared with 95% (38 of 40) of controls. Unfortunately, this study suffered from two major drawbacks. First, the studied interval was only eight days and therefore has little relevance to the clinical situation. Second, the infected pouch model employed in this experiment is seriously flawed. This is due to the unpredictable effects of systemic clearance and recirculation of the infecting organisms, as well as the inevitable equilibrium established between the soaked prosthesis and the surrounding tissues. Nonetheless, this early report suggested the possibility of passively imparting antimicrobial resistance to a prosthetic vascular graft.

Several in vitro studies have attempted to select the most effective antibiotic to absorb onto a graft in a passive system. In one report by Powell et al, several antibiotics were studied to determine their duration of antimicrobial activity following passive soaking in an in vivo elution model.[20] Tested agents included: a) oxacillin; b) first, second and third generation cephalosporins; c) the aminoglycosides tobramycin and gentamicin; d) tetracycline; and e) rifampin. Each antibiotic was added to an aliquot of blood used to preclot an 8 mm Dacron prosthesis. Treated and control grafts were then implanted into canine infrarenal aortas and exposed to arterial flow for up to 24 hours. Graft rings were removed and tested for antimicrobial activity at intervals of 0 minutes, 15 minutes, 60 minutes and 24 hours. At 24 hours, only those grafts preclotted with blood containing rifampin disclosed any measurable activity. At this interval, rifampin soaked grafts retained 91% of their original activity. In our laboratory, we have confirmed the superiority

Table 1. Table shows reported methods of bonding antibiotics to prosthetic vascular grafts.

Bond Type	Author	Year	Graft	Antibiotic	Bonding Agent
Passive	Richardson et al[19]	1970	Dacron	Cephalothin	None
	Powell et al[20]	1983	Dacron	Rifampin	Clotted Blood
	McDougal et al[21]	1986	Dacron	Rifampin	Clotted Blood
	Goëau-Brissonnière et al[22]	1991	Dacron	rifampin	Gelatin
	Avramovic et al[23]	1992	Dacron	Rifampin	Gelatin
Topical	Shenk et al[13]	1989	PTFE	Tobramycin	NBCA
	Ney et al[15]	1990	PTFE	Tobramycin	Fibrin
	Haverich et al[25]	1992	Dacron	Gentamicin	Fibrin
Ionic	Clark et al[29]	1974	Dacron	Silver	Allantoin
	Prahlad et al[7]	1981	PTFE	Penicillin G	BC
	Henry et al[8]	1981	PTFE	Oxacillin Penicillin G	BC
	Greco et al[9]	1982	PTFE	Oxacillin	BC
	Harvey et al[11]	1982	PTFE	Penicillin G	TDMAC
	Greco et al[10]	1984	PTFE	Cefoxitin	TDMAC
	Benvenisty et al[4]	1986	PTFE	Amikacin Oxacillin	AgNO_3
	Modak et al[5]	1987	Dacron PTFE	Norfloxacin Oxacillin	TDMAC AgNO_3
	Shue et al[12]	1988	Dacron	Oxacillin	TDMAC
	Kinney et al[6]	1991	PTFE	Ciprofloxacin	TDMAC AgNO_3
Retention	Moore et al[16]	1981	Dacron	Amikacin	Collagen
	Sobinsky et al[14]	1986	PTFE	Cefoxitin	GK
	Chervu et al[17]	1991	Dacron	Rifampin	Collagen
	Colburn et al[28]	1992	Dacron	Rifampin	Collagen

PTFE - Polytetrafluoroethylene, NBCA - N-butyl-2-cyanoacrylate
BC - Benzalkonium chloride, TDMAC - Tridodecylmethyl-ammonium chloride
AgNO_3 - Silver nitrate, GK - Glucosaminoglycan-keratin

of rifampin compared to either amikacin or chloramphenicol when mixed with blood and used to preclot Dacron grafts.[17] The greater persistence of antimicrobial activity in grafts passively soaked with rifampin, compared to other agents, is presumably related to the hydrophobic properties of this compound.

The ability of rifampin, applied passively to a prosthetic graft, to protect against infection has been studied experimentally in vivo by several investigators. In 1986, McDougal and associates implanted Dacron grafts, preclotted with blood mixed with rifampin, into the aortas of dogs.[21] The grafts were subsequently challenged with an intravenous infusion of 10^7 organisms of *Staphylococcus aureus* immediately postoperatively. After three weeks, the grafts were removed, cultured and compared to identically processed control untreated grafts. The results demonstrated that none (0 of 5) of the rifampin protected grafts were infected where as 3 of 5 control grafts were culture positive. It is not clear whether these results would be duplicated had the bacterial challenge not been given in the immediate postoperative period. This is due to the fact that, although passive soaking has been shown to impart antimicrobial activity to a prosthetic graft, the long-term duration of this protection is questionable.

Two recent studies have appeared in the literature examining the ability of protein-sealed Dacron grafts, protected with rifampin, to prevent vascular graft infection. The first study was reported by Goëau-Brissonnière and associates in 1991.[22] In this study, antibiotic bonding was obtained by soaking gelatin-sealed Dacron grafts in a 1 mg/ml rifampin solution for 15 minutes. Uncoated control, untreated gelatin-sealed and rifampin soaked gelatin-sealed grafts were then used for a thoracoabdominal aortic bypass performed in dogs. Two days following insertion of the grafts, 5×10^5 colony forming units (CFU) of *Staphylococcus aureus* were administered intravenously. All grafts were harvested five days later and submitted for analysis of bacterial counts. Both uncoated and untreated gelatin-sealed Dacron grafts were culture positive in 100% (6 of 6) of cases. On the other hand, no (0 of 6) rifampin treated graft was infected. In a related study, Avramovic et al recently reported their results using a gelatin-sealed Dacron graft passively soaked with rifampin.[23] For this experiment, both treated and untreated grafts were inserted into the carotid arteries of sheep. Prior to closing the wounds, each graft was contaminated by the direct inoculation of 10^8 CFU of *Staphylococcus aureus.* After three weeks the grafts were removed and cultured. The results again favored the rifampin treated prostheses with only 2 of 10 grafts testing culture positive compared to 6 of 8 survivors in the control group. As with previous studies, neither of these experiments address the ability of a passively bonded prosthesis to prevent infection following a late bacterial challenge. Also, it should be mentioned that the soaking of a protein-sealed Dacron graft in a rifampin solution likely results in a different chemical bond than the passive absorption of the same antibiotic onto an uncoated graft. The negatively changed carboxyl groups found on the gelatin sealant may bond to the positively changed rifampin molecules. Therefore, these two experiments in which gelatin-sealed Dacron prostheses were studied may be more correctly compared to the reports using ionic bonding methods described below.

TOPICAL APPLICATION

Three papers reporting the protection of vascular grafts by the topical application of antibiotic sealants have previously been published. The earliest description of this technique came in a report by Shenk et al in 1988.[13] In this experiment, the chemical glue *N*-butyl-2-cyanoacrylate was used as an adhesive vehicle to bind tobramycin to the external surface of PTFE grafts. The protocol studied the efficacy of this suspension in both a canine direct contamination model and following the replacement of a previously infected PTFE graft. In both cases, the protection afforded by the application of the tobramycin sealant was highly statistically significant. Unfortunately, the cyanoacrylate glues have been reported to be highly toxic compounds and their routine use in humans requires caution.[24] To avoid the issue of tissue toxicity, the endogenous protein fibrin has been advocated as a substitute glue for the topical application of antibiotics to vascular grafts. Ney and associates first reported the use of a fibrin/antibiotic suspension for this purpose.[15] In this study PTFE grafts, contaminated with a solution containing 3×10^8 CFU of both *Escherichia coli* and *Staphylococcus aureus*, were implanted into canine aortas. Animals were then divided into three groups: those which received no therapy, those that were sealed with fibrin only without antibiotics, and lastly a group of dogs in which the contaminated graft was sealed with a fibrin/tobramycin suspension. By the fourth postoperative day, all animals in both control groups either died or had to be reoperated on because of graft sepsis. Furthermore, all of these grafts were found to be culture positive. The animals in the experimental fibrin+antibiotic group all survived until 17 days following graft implantation when they were sacrificed. However, although all these experimental grafts had normal anastomoses, three out of four grafts were found to have positive cultures. Most recently, Haverich and associates reported their results using a Dacron prosthesis protected with a sealant derived from the combination of fibrin and gentamicin.[25] Preliminary in vitro elution studies using this system documented retained antibiotic activity for up to 21 days. Unfortunately, the in vivo experimental protocol, which utilized both control and experimental graft segments in the same animal, makes interpretation of the results of this study quite difficult.

Direct Ionic Bonding

Experiments examining the possibility of ionic bonding of antibiotics to a prosthetic vascular graft have primarily focused on the use of two bonding agents: benzalkonium chloride and TDMAC. Most of the early work using the surfactant benzalkonium chloride was performed by Greco and his associates.[7-9,18] In this method, a positively charged penicillin antibiotic (either penicillin G or oxacillin) is applied to the surface of a PTFE graft by ionic bonding to the negatively charged surfactant. Two early studies documented the efficacy of this technique in vivo in a infected subcutaneous pouch model.[7,8] Since this time, several studies have also shown this method to be effective when used as bypass grafts in the aortic position.[9,18]

TDMAC is a quarternary ammonium salt with three negatively charged alkyl side groups and has been shown to be up to five times more effective in bonding positively charged antibiotics to prosthetic graft surfaces.[10] Several reports documenting the ability of TDMAC to protect both PTFE and Dacron grafts form infection have appeared in the literature.[5,6,11,12] In the most recent report, Kinney and associates studied PTFE grafts bonded with a TDMAC/ciprofloxacin combination.[6] In this study, the authors demonstrated that this combination provided an effective source of local antibiotic release at high levels for up to 14 days.

Retention

Two biological proteins have been studied for their ability to retain antibiotics on a vascular graft: glucosaminoglycan-keratin and collagen. The combination of glucosaminoglycan and keratin proteins forms a biodegradable solution that is capable of binding antibiotics to prosthetic surfaces. The first report, utilizing this method for the protection of a vascular graft was made by Sobinsky and associates.[14] In this study, control and treated PTFE grafts were implanted into canine common carotid arteries. Treated grafts were protected by a combination of glucosaminoglycan-keratin and cefoxitin. Immediately following graft implantation, the animals were challenged with an intravenous infusion of

10^8 organisms of *Staphylococcus aureus*. Grafts were removed and cultured at ten different intervals between 1 and 28 days postinfusion. Results demonstrated that while 100% (10 of 10) of the unprotected grafts were infected, only 1 of 10 treated grafts was culture positive.

The use of collagen as bonding agent in an antibiotic delivery system was first reported by Krajicek et al in 1969.[26] Since that time, our laboratory has gained considerable experience using this technique. To test the hypothesis that a collagen/antibiotic release system could provide prolonged antimicrobial activity, we have utilized an in vitro elution system. Graft samples, 6 mm in diameter, are placed into a flask containing 250 ml of 5% albumen and continually agitated. The fluid in the flask is totally removed and replaced every 24 hours. Two graft disk samples are removed from the flask each day and placed on a blood agar plate infected with *Staphylococcus aureus*. The zones of inhibition found on each plate are then measured and recorded daily. Samples are studied until no bacteriostatic effect is noted. Utilizing this system, the following experiment was performed. Amikacin, chloramphenicol and rifampin were bonded to double velour Dacron grafts with minimally cross-linked type 1 collagen.[17] A fourth experiment in which a graft without collagen was preclotted with blood mixed with rifampin was also tested. Each graft was tested at daily intervals in our bioassay for anti-staphylococcal activity after continuous elution in the in vitro agitation system. The results demonstrated that the collagen bonded graft impregnated with rifampin was superior to either amikacin or chloramphenicol and had an overall duration of activity of 22 days. In addition, rifampin alone without collagen, although not as effective as the collagen bonded rifampin graft, was superior to both amikacin and chloramphenicol when mixed with blood and used to pre-clot the graft. This finding confirms the results reported by Powell et al, in which grafts demonstrated prolonged antimicrobial activity after being pre-clotted with blood containing rifampin.[20]

The ability of the rifampin impregnated collagen graft to prevent infection in vivo has been studied in two separate experiments. The first experiment was designed to examine the resistance of this graft to a bacteremic challenge as a function of time following implantation.[27] Fifty 6-mm Dacron grafts, impregnated with either collagen (control) or collagen plus rifampin (experimental), were implanted end-to-end into the infrarenal aorta. The retroperitoneum and abdominal wall were closed, in layers and the animals allowed to recover. The dogs were then divided into four groups; each with an experimental and control arm. At 2, 7, 10 or 12 days after graft implantation, sequential groups were challenged with 1.2×10^8 organisms of *Staphylococcus aureus* intravenously. Three weeks after this hematogenous seeding, the grafts were harvested. Control and experimental grafts were compared by evaluating patency and culture proven infection as a function of implantation time prior to the bacteremic challenge. Three dogs died after bacterial infusion and were excluded from further analysis. The results of this study showed that collagen coated grafts could be infected up to seven days after implantation. After seven days, it appeared that healing of the collagen graft surface interferes with delayed bacterial seeding. The experimental rifampin impregnated graft could not be infected when challenged up to seven days after implant. At 10 and 12 days, one graft and two grafts respectively had positive cultures in the experimental group. Therefore, this study indicated that a vascular prostheses, protected with rifampin in a collagen release system, could maintain prolonged resistance to infection in a challenging bacteremic model.

Having demonstrated that the rifampin impregnated collagen graft was effective in resisting infection when challenged intravenously, a second experiment was performed to test whether this ability extended to a bacterial challenge by direct contamination.[28] In this study, experimental antibiotic protected grafts were implanted in situ into a previously infected aortic bed. Eighty-three adult mongrel dogs underwent implantation of a 3 cm untreated Dacron graft into the infrarenal aorta. This initial graft was deliberately infected, at the time of operation, with 10^2 organisms of *Staphylococcus aureus* by direct inoculation. One week later, the dogs were re-explored, the retroperitoneum debrided and the animals randomized to undergo an end-to-end graft replacement with either one of two types of prosthetic grafts: Group I (Collagen, n=36) received control collagen impregnated knitted Dacron grafts, Group II (rifampin, n=47) received experimental collagen-rifampin bonded Dacron grafts. Each group of animals was then subdivided to receive one of four treatment protocols: a) no antibiotic therapy (No Abx), b) cephalosporin peritoneal irrigation solution (cefazolin 500 mg/1000 cc) during surgery and two doses of cephalosporin (cefazolin, 500 mg IM) postoperatively (Peri-op), c) Peri-op plus one week of cephalosporin (cefazolin, 500 mg IM, BID) (One wk) and d) Peri-op plus two weeks of cephalosporin (cefazolin, 500 mg IM, BID) (two weeks). All grafts were sterilely removed 4 weeks after implantation. There were no anastomotic disruptions and all grafts were patent at the time of removal. Cultures were obtained from the grafts and perigraft tissues separately. Analysis included determination of the culture status (positive or negative) of tissue and graft samples combined (T&G Cx), as well as of the graft segments alone (Graft Cx) irrespective of the results of the surrounding tissue cultures. Results were expressed as the percentage of animals which were culture positive at sacrifice. In all four treatment groups the reduction of positive graft cultures (Graft Cx), following replacement of a previously infected aortic prosthesis with a collagen-rifampin bonded graft, was statistically significant. When overall infection rates (T&G Cx) are evaluated, this reduction was statistically significant only in the subset of animals treated with two weeks of supplemental antibiotics. In conclusion, it appears that the collagen-rifampin bonded graft reduces the incidence of graft colonization following replacement of an infected graft. However, a course of supplemental antibiotics is required to sterilize the surrounding perigraft tissues.

In summary, the available experimental evidence clearly suggests that a Dacron vascular prosthesis, impregnated with rifampin using a collagen release system, is effective in resisting contamination in a canine model. Also, results following an in situ reconstruction using this graft have been encouraging. Whether this laboratory data will translate into any clinical benefit must await the completion of properly performed randomized controlled clinical trials.

REFERENCES

1. Malone JM, Moore WS, Campagna G, Bean B. Bacteremic infectability of vascular grafts: The influence of pseudointimal integrity and duration of graft infection. Surgery 1975; 78: 211-216.
2. Goldstone J, Moore WS. Infection in vascular prostheses: clinical manifestations and surgical management. Am J Surg 1974; 128: 225-233.
3. Fry WJ, Lindenauer SM. Infection complicating the use of plastic arterial implants. Arch Surg 1967; 94: 600-609.
4. Benvenisty A, Tannenbaum G, Ahlborn TN et al. Control of prosthetic bacterial infection: evaluation of an easily incorporated, tightly bound, silver antibiotic PTFE graft. J Surg Res 1986; 44: 1-7.
5. Modak SM, Sampath L, Fox CL et al. A new method for the direct incorporation of antibiotic in prosthetic vascular grafts. Surg Gynecol Obstet 1987; 164: 143-147.
6. Kinney EV, Bandyk DF, Seabrook GA et al. Antibiotic-bonded PTFE vascular grafts: the effect of silver antibiotic on bioactivity following implantation. J Surg Res 1991; 50: 430-435.
7. Prahlad A, Harvey RA, Greco RS. Diffusion of antibiotics from a polytetrafluoroethylene-benzalkonium surface. Am Surg 1981; 47: 515-518.
8. Henry R, Harvey RA, Greco RS. Antibiotic bonding to vascular prostheses. J Thorac Cardiovasc Surg 1981; 82: 272-277.
9. Greco RS, Harvey RA, Smilow PC, Tesoriero JV. Prevention of vascular prosthetic infection by a benzalkonium-oxacillin bonded polytetrafluoroethylene graft. Surg Gynecol Obstet 1982; 155: 28-32.

10. Greco RS, Harvey RA. The biochemical bonding of cefoxitin to a microporous polytetrafluoroethylene surface. J Surg Res 1984; 36: 237-243.
11. Harvey RA, Alcid DV, Greco RS. Antibiotic bonding to polytetrafluoroethylene with tridodecylmethylammonium chloride. Surgery 1982; 92(3): 504-512.
12. Shue WB, Worosilo SC, Donetz AP et al. Prevention of vascular prosthetic infection with an antibiotic-bonded Dacron graft. J Vasc Surg 1988; 8: 600-605.
13. Shenk JS, Ney AL, Tsukayama DT et al. Tobramycin-adhesive in preventing and treating PTFE vascular graft infections. J Surg Res 1989; 47: 487-492.
14. Sobinsky KR, Flanigan DP. Antibiotic binding to polytetrafluoroethylene via glucosaminoglycan-keratin luminal coating. Surgery 1986; 100(4): 629-634.
15. Ney AL, Kelly PH, Tsukayama DT, Bubrick MP. Fibrin glue-antibiotic suspension in the prevention of prosthetic graft infection. J Trauma 1990; 30(8): 1000-1006.
16. Moore WS, Chvapil M, Sieffert G, Keown K. Development of an infection resistant vascular prosthesis. Arch Surg 1981; 116: 1403-1407.
17. Chervu A, Moore WS, Chvapil M, Henderson T. Efficacy and duration of antistaphylococcal activity comparing three antibiotics bonded to Dacron vascular grafts with a collagen release system. J Vasc Surg 1991; 13: 897-901.
18. Greco RS, Harvey RA. The role of antibiotic bonding in the prevention of vascular prosthetic infections. Ann Surg 1982; 195(2): 168-171.
19. Richardson RL, Pate JW, Wolf RY et al. The outcome of antibiotic-soaked arterial grafts in guinea pig wounds contaminated with *E. coli* or *S. aureus.* J Thor Cardiovasc Surg 1970; 59: 635-637.
20. Powell TW, Burnham SJ, Johnson G. A passive system using rifampin to create an infection-resistant vascular prosthesis. Surgery 1983; 94(5): 765-769.
21. McDougal EG, Burnham SJ, Johnson G. Rifampin protection against experimental graft sepsis. J Vasc Surg 1986; 4: 5-7.
22. Goëau-Brissonnière O, Leport C, Bascourt F et al. Prevention of vascular graft infection by rifampin bonding to a gelatin-sealed Dacron graft. Ann Vasc Surg 1991; 5: 408-412.
23. Avramovic J, Fletcher JP. Prevention of prosthetic vascular graft infection by rifampicin impregnation of a protein-sealed Dacron graft in combination with parenteral cephalosporin. J Cardiovasc Surg 1992; 33: 70-74.
24. Lehman R, West R, Leonard F. Toxicity of alkyl-2-cyanoacrylates. Arch Surg 1966; 93: 447.
25. Haverich A, Hirt S, Karek M et al. Prevention of graft infection by bonding of gentamycin to Dacron prostheses. J Vasc Surg 1992; 15: 187-193.
26. Krajicek M, Dvorak J, Chvapil M. Infection-resistant synthetic vascular substitutes. J Cardiovasc Surg 1969; 10: 454.
27. Chervu A, Moore WS, Gelabert HA et al. Prevention of graft infection by use of prostheses bonded with a rifampin/collagen release system. J Vasc Surg 1991; 14(4): 521-525.
28. Colburn MD, Moore WS, Gelabert HA et al. Use of an antibiotic-bonded graft for in-situ reconstruction following prosthetic graft infections. J Vasc Surg 1992; : .
29. Clark RE, Margraf HW. Antibacterial vascular grafts with improved thromboresistance. Arch Surg 1974; 109: 159-162.

CHAPTER 7

FUTURE DIRECTIONS IN THE DEVELOPMENT OF BACTERIAL RESISTANT GRAFTS

George E. Hajjar
Hugh A. Gelabert

INTRODUCTION

Despite major advances in vascular grafting, since the original publication in 1952 on the use of Vinyon-N, the currently available synthetic vascular grafts fall short of fulfilling all the desired criteria for the ideal graft. This chapter deals with the various attempts at developing a vascular substitute that would be capable of resisting graft infection and speculates on some theoretical developments that might be pursued in the future in order to achieve this goal and prevent this disastrous complication in vascular surgery. Such an endeavor could be achieved by approaching the problem from various angles: improving graft material, improving graft healing and developing a more specific and efficient antibiotic delivery system.

GRAFT MATERIAL

The synthetic vascular grafts currently in use are perceived as foreign bodies, and as such they carry the associated risk of infection which is hard to eradicate once the graft is contaminated. The use of arterial homografts was abandoned due to rejection and degeneration.

The development of an experimental bioresorbable vascular graft by Greisler and his colleagues opened a new horizon in the search for the ideal graft.[1] A graft that would act as a temporary matrix and gradually be resorbed and replaced by newly synthesized and totally biogenic material and thus would be theoretically, infection resistant. Such polyglicolic acid (PGA) grafts were tested on rabbits and found to be resorbed between four weeks and three months following implantation. There were no hemorrhagic complications seen, but the rate of aneurysm formation was 10% and distal anastomotic stenosis 15%. The (PGA) prosthesis was digested by macrophages and giant cells and replaced by an outer capsule of fibroblasts. The inner capsule consisted of myofibroblasts and endothelial cells possibly originating from transinterstitial capillary ingrowth. No such prosthesis is yet available for clinical use. The problem of aneurysm formation is being studied and could possibly be overcome by the use of semiresorbable material or a mixture of substances that would resorb at different rates. This would allow capsule and neointima formation, while the slower resorbing substance provides a mechanical strut while maturation occurs.

Another concept in the development of infection resistant grafts is the use of allografts. With cryopreservation techniques and the development of new generation anti-rejection drugs this should minimize the problem of degeneration. Early work on such a graft has been performed by Moore and his colleagues who used these grafts for arterial reconstruction in an infected field.[2] These investigators used human aortic grafts which had been preserved by simple freezing. These grafts were subsequently implanted in infected aortic fields. The principal problem with these large caliber grafts was the tendency to develop aneurysmal degeneration over the course of time. The conclusion of these investigators was these grafts represented a promising avenue of investigation, but that the tendency of pseudoaneurysmal degeneration limited their long term use. Other investigators have maintained interest in this field by varying the method of preserving the graft and studying the immunological characteristics of allografts.[3,4] Perhaps the most promising development was the advance of improved preservation techniques based on the use of DMSO and cell growth media.[5]

More recent work in this area has been presented by Berman and colleagues.[6] They demonstrated the successful use of cryopreserved grafts in the construction of A-V fistulas. They noted that the preservation techniques involved the presoaking of the grafts in a solution of DMSO, fetal calf serum and RPMI. The grafts were then slowly frozen and preserved in a tissue bank until needed. The clinical use of these small caliber grafts in instances of infection and accelerated intimal hyperplastic occlusion revealed reasonable function at 12 to 18 months. The persistent problem of pseudoaneusymal degeneration required reinforcing some grafts with a PTFE mesh.

GRAFT HEALING

Graft healing occurs via two mechanisms. Transanastomotic pannus growth and transinterstitial neointimal formation. The latter only seen in laboratory studies and yet to be reported in humans. The neointima that lines the blood contacting surface of the graft in humans consists of a compacted fibrin coagulum. Only for a short distance from the anastomosis does the neointima formed contain endothelial cells. Graft healing could be promoted by binding a stimulator of cell migration and proliferation to the implanted graft. Early coverage of the graft by the neointima will provide a smooth surface and afford protection against bacterial seeding. Such grafts have been developed and experimentally tested in a canine model by Greisler and his colleagues at Loyola University. Their grafts bonded to endothelial cell growth factor (ECGF) demonstrated enhancement of capillary ingrowth and a more complete reendothelilization compared to the nonbonded grafts.[7]

Endothelial cell seeding of newly implanted vascular prostheses was introduced experimentally in an attempt to decrease the thrombogenicity of synthetic grafts.[8,9,10] Only few studies have been published on its clinical efficacy in increasing patency rates in small diameter 6-8 mm prostheses.[11] Theoretically it not only improves patency rates but should provide a more complete and earlier coverage of the graft surface, forming a barrier to bacterial seeding of the graft in the early postoperative period. Such a study has not been published, but experimental work showed that seeded grafts did have endothelial cell patches as early as four days postimplantation, and at four months endothelialization was 100%. The nonseeded grafts on the other hand, still showed areas containing red thrombus and fibrin up to one year postimplantation.[9,12]

ANTIBIOTIC BONDING TO GRAFTS

Historically, attempts to impregnate and bind antibiotics to grafts have used a variety of chemical and mechanical techniques to accomplish their goal. These have included passive soaking of grafts in antibiotic solutions, ionic bonding of the antibiotic to the graft and covalent bonding of the antibiotic to an electrostatically charged graft.

Subsequent developments include the binding of antibiotics by mechanical inclusion within a degradable protein film which is applied to the prosthetic graft. These so-called retention bonding methods have been described by Moore and his associates in the development of their rifampin inpregnated grafts.[13] In essence, the rifampin is captured within interstices of the collagen coating of their graft, it is thus mechanically retained until protein degradation releases the antibiotic. By this method, the duration of the antibiotic activity should be proportional to the relative concentration of collagen and antibiotic and the amount of collagen/antibiotic mixture applied to the graft.

Most recently the bonding of rifampin and collagen grafts has been accomplished by a method referred to as pH shifting. In essence, the collagen-coated graft is immersed into a mildly acidic solution which allows diffusion of the rifampin into the collagen matrix. The graft is then soaked in an alkaline solution which has the effect of stabilizing the rifampin within the graft. This technique has the advantages of being relatively inexpensive and simple. The method has not been extensively tested, and to date does not appear superior to the previously noted collagen bonded rifampin graft.

Retention of the antibiotic activity has been one of the long-standing problems in the development of antibiotic bonded grafts. Improved methods of binding antibiotics to grafts have resulted in extending the duration of antibiotic activity to approximately 21 days following implantation.[14] After this point, the antibiotic bound to the graft is usually depleted, and the graft reverts to an unprotected state. Should a patient experience an event which would be considered to place his graft at increased risk of infection, oral prophylactic antibiotics are recommended. Oral antibiotics lack specificity and cannot be targeted. Thus despite an adequate dose, the actual concentration of antibiotic in the region of the graft is quite low. One idea proposed to increase the concentration of the antibiotics in the area of the graft is to direct the antibiotic activity by binding with antibodies. If the antibiotic could be bound to an antibody specifically targeted against the graft then the graft could be repeatedly covered with antibiotic. This has raised the notion of "recharging" a graft's antibiotic activity as needed in various clinical situations. While this idea remains speculative, the same concept has been applied in the areas of oncology and transplantation as means of specifically identifying and targeting a variety of cell lines.

THE IDEAL GRAFT

The concept of an ideal graft has undergone gradual transformation over the course of the last 30 years. Initially, an ideal graft was thought to be one which could hold blood and was available off the shelf. The definition of an ideal graft has advanced. Subsequent requirements for an ideal graft include thromboresistance, infection resistance, compliance matching, longevity, lack of immunogenicity or toxicity.

THE BIOSYNTHETIC GRAFT

A relatively recent description of an ideal graft noted the concept of melding both biological and prosthetic materials into a biosynthetic graft.[15] This graft was conceived as taking advantage of the best features of both the synthetic grafts and the biological conduits. Such grafts would contain all the elements constituting the vessel wall including endothelial cells, smooth muscle cells and fibroblasts. These would be placed on a synthetic graft which would provide structural integrity and longevity.

THE GENETICALLY ENGINEERED GRAFT

More recent notions of an idealized graft include genetic modulation of endothelial cells. In this effort the modulation is directed towards enhancing some endothelial functions, suppressing other functions and adding characteristics which may not belong to the cell line or even the organism. Specific interventions could include the enhancement of thrombolytic functions or anticoagulative functions such as the expression of tissue plasminogen activator or heparinoid activity. Another variation includes the inhibition of cellular replication and matrix excretion in order to inhibit intimal hyperplasia. With regards to bacterial resistance, the insertion of genetic instructions for the production of glycoproteins and antibiotics could conceivably alter the susceptibility of the grafts to bacterial infection.

Whether these endothelial cells are carried in an autogenous vein, a homologous vein or even a xenograft vein remains to be established. Alternative notions include the construction of a prosthetic matrix upon which the endothelial cells are seeded or the construction of a biosynthetic matrix upon which to seed the endothelium. Both these projects are under development but have not approached clinical use. Finally, the concept of a totally synthetic biological graft has arisen where all elements of a graft would be grown in tissue cultures and layered onto one another in order to recreate a blood vessel.

CONCLUSION

The field of infection-resistant grafts has generated considerable interest and research. While the problem of graft infection is relatively uncommon, the consequences of these infections has pressed the demand for improved grafts. While several antibiotic bonded grafts have been developed, none has seen clinical application in humans. The pace of advances in this area would lead to the expectation that some form of clinically useful application of this technique would be forthcoming soon. Over the long-term, the prospects for an advanced biosynthetic graft are very good. Until such a time, meticulous sterile technique, perioperative antibiotics and pharmacological control of coagulation will remain the standards of care.

REFERENCES

1. Greisler HP. Arterial regeneration over absorbable prostheses. Arch Surg 1982; 177: 1425-1431.
2. Moore WS, Swanson RJ, Campagna G et al. The use of fresh tissue arterial substitutes in infected fields. J Surg Res 1975; 18: 229-234.
3. Piccone V, Sika J, Ahmed N et al. Preserved saphenous vein allografts for vascular access. Surg Gynecol Obstet 1978; 147: 385-90.
4. Perloff L, Beckard C, Rowlands D, Barker C. The venous homograft: An immunological question. Surgery 1972; 72: 961-70.
5. Ladin D, Lindenauer S, Burkel W et al. Viability, immunogenic reaction and patency of cryopreserves venous allografts. Surg Forum 1982; 33: 460-63.
6. Berman S, Glickman M, Hurwitz R et al. Cryopreserved human saphenous vein allografts and their use in construction of chronic hemodialysis access. In: Sommer BG, Henry ML, ed. Vascular access for hemodialysis. Chicago: Pluribus Press, 1991: 219-228.
7. Greisler HP, Klosak J, Dennis JW et al. Biomaterial pretreatment with ECGF to augment endothelial cell proliferation. J Vasc Surg 1987; 2: 393-402.
8. Herring M, Gardner A, Glover J. A single-staged technique for seeding vascular grafts with autogenous endothelium. Surgery 1978; 84: 498-504.
9. Graham LM, Burkel WE, Stanley JC. Immediate seeding of enzymatically derived endothelium in Dacron vascular grafts. Arch Surg 1982; 115: 1269-1294.
10. Sharefkin JB, Latker CH, D'Amore PA et al. Seeding of Dacron vascular prostheses with endothelium of aortic origin. J Surg Res 1980; 34: 33-43.

11. Herring M, Gardner A, Glover J. Seeding human arterial prosthesis with mechanically derived endothelium. Detrimental effect of smoking. J Vasc Surg 1984; 2: 278-279.
12. Burkel WE, Ford JW, Vinter DW et al. Sequential studies of healing in endothelial seeded vascular prostheses: Histologic and ultrastructure characteristics of vascular incorporation. J Surg Res 1981; 30: 305-324.
13. Moore WS, Chvapil M, Seiffert G, Keown K. Development of an infection-resistant vascular prosthesis. Arch Surg 1981; 116: 1403-1407.
14. Chervu A, Moore WS, Chvapil M, Henderson T. Efficacy and duration of antistaphylococcal activity comparing three antibiotics bonded to Dacron vascular grafts with a collagen release system. J Vasc Surg 1991; 13: 897-901.
15. Moore WS. The ideal vascular substitute. In: Skotnicki B, Reinaerts, ed. Recent advances in vascular grafting. Gerrards Cross, Buckinghamshire, England: System 4 Associates, 1984: 282-284.

INDEX